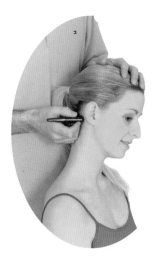

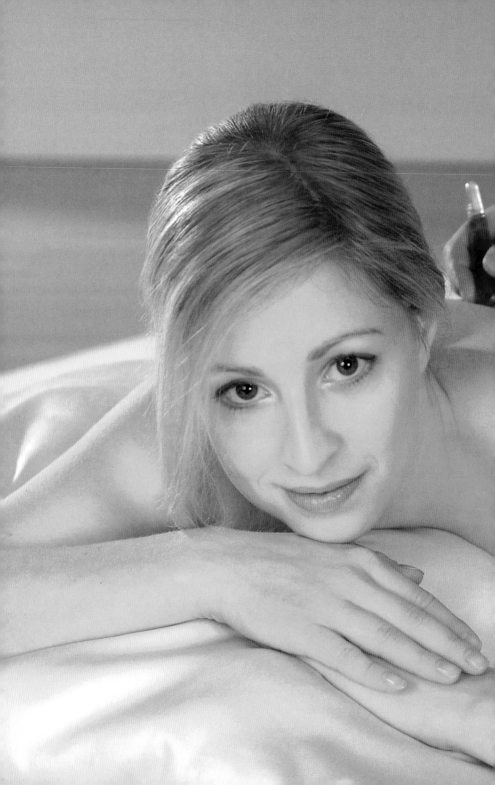

Ewald Kliegel

Crystal
Wands

*For healing,
massage therapy
and reflexology*

Photography by
Ines Blersch

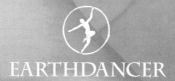

EARTHDANCER

A FINDHORN PRESS IMPRINT

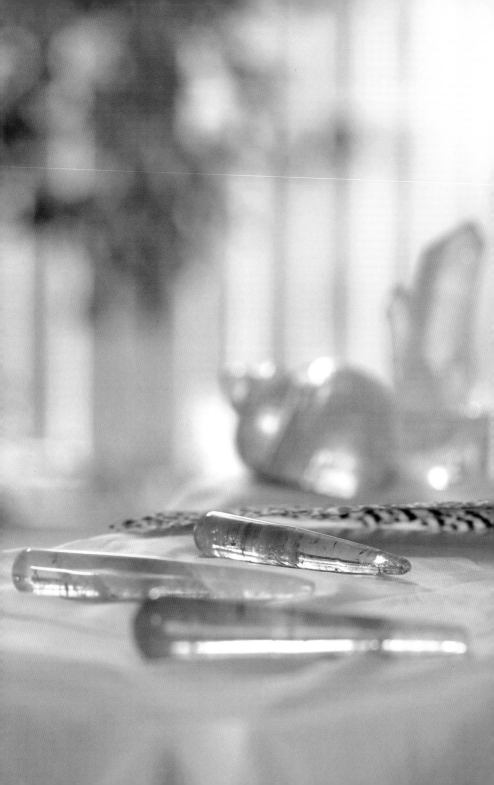

Contents

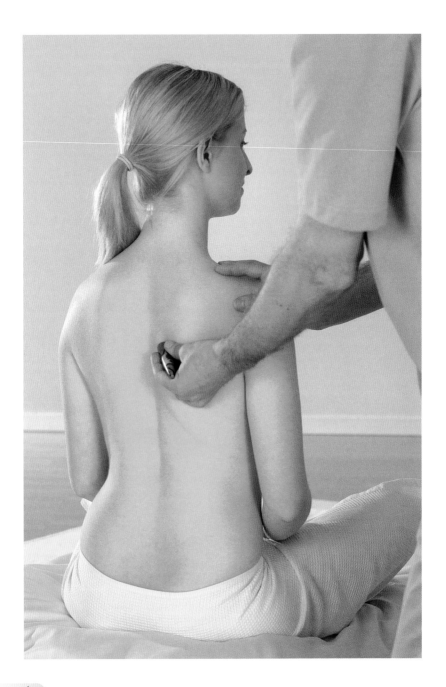

Introduction

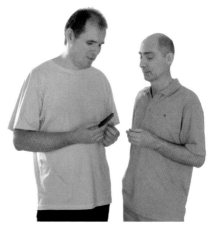

Michael Gienger and Ewald Kliegel

Just imagine ... something exists that you can easily do to create a sense of wellbeing and good health in others, something suited to virtually every situation, something small children enjoy and sportspeople value, something that is in the service of Love...

These are bold claims. But all of them can be achieved, very simply, through massage with crystal wands.

Using crystal wands to support the process of massage, for reflexology, to trace meridian lines, to balance the chakras – whatever your treatment therapy, crystal wands will help you.

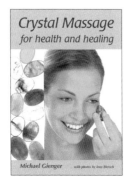

Crystal Massage for Health and Healing, published in 2006,* introduces the basic methods of applying crystals for massage. Since its publication, interest in the methods has grown to such an extent that additional information has been written on each individual method. Massage with crystal wands is the topic for discussion in this book, and adds to the growing body of information on the use of crystals for massage.

The story of crystal wands began in 1996 during a conversation in Michael Gienger's summer garden. We had met that day to discuss ways of making our treatments more effective. On the one

Michael Gienger, *Crystal Massage for Health and Healing*, Earthdancer a Findhorn Press Imprint hand we had reflexology, which had been tried and tested for many years, and which had obtained an additional positive quality through the use of crystals. On the other hand, we wanted to use our growing knowledge and experience of those crystalline mineral treasures of the Earth more intensely for direct physical contact. At the time, we a procedure that combines in itself many new departure points.

The round end of the crystal wand can be used almost like a crystal sphere in massage, and the pointed end can be used to target acupressure points or to trace meridian lines. In addition, by means of brief pre-testing procedures, it is also possible to identify a suitable

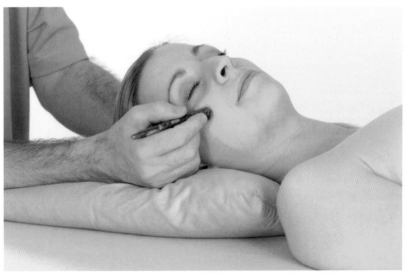

Crystal Wands for Massage

already had considerable experience with the use of tumbled stones and spheres, had applied crystals by laying them on, and had carried out energetic treatments. All of those methods continue to be sought after. However, the new element in all this was the use of crystal *wands*, crystal wand for a particular treatment or application. Massages thus become indisputably more effective.

Combined efforts over the years have borne fruit, and massage with crystals now has a firm and growing place in the fields of wellness and

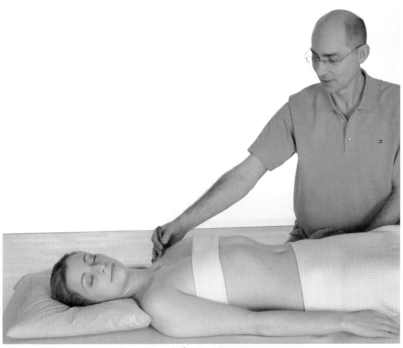

Crystal Wands for Meridian Treatments

therapy. Both Crystal Balance® and the gem oils developed by Monika Grundmann* are creating new paths in cosmetics and wellness, the Aurum Manus® treatments by Ricky Welch** are recognised as tinnitus and migraine therapies, whilst the popularity of the Joya® massage roller invented by Ulrich Metz has spread across Europe like wildfire. These are but a few of the many examples of successes made possible through treatments with crystals over the last few years.

I would now like to introduce to you the beautiful and fascinating possibility of bestowing a sense of wellbeing and good health with crystal wands.

Autumn 2007
Ewald Kliegel

* Monika Grundmann, *Crystal Balance*, Earthdancer a Findhorn Press Imprint, 2008
** Ricky Welch, *Aurum Manus*, Earthdancer a Findhorn Press Imprint, 2006

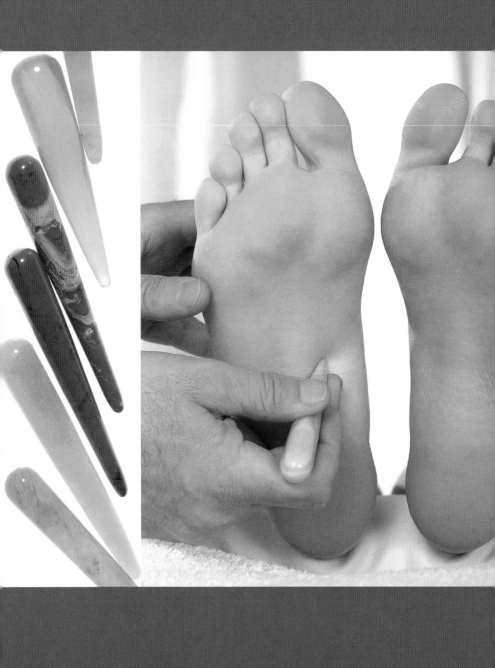

Basics

Do Crystal Wands Really Work?

'What difference does it make whether I carry out a massage with or without crystal wands?' 'Do they actually work?' These are the two questions I hear most often in connection with crystal wands. You can find answers to both questions quite easily by carrying out a simple test on yourself. Everyone's head has reflexology zones, which are responsible for good blood circulation in the feet. People with cold feet (usually women) may experience a clear improvement via those zones. Just do this simple little test:

First massage the zones shown in the figure below for about 2-3 minutes with your fingers. Then repeat the massage about a quarter of an hour later with a crystal wand made of Rock Crystal, Amethyst, Chalcedony or Sodalite. Finally, massage these zones again half an hour later with a Snowflake Obsidian crystal wand.

Experience has shown that a massage using Snowflake Obsidian causes the feet to feel warmer soonest. If you try this application again on another occasion and change the sequence, you are certain to achieve the best success with the Snowflake Obsidian.

The test demonstrates that your choice of crystal wand clearly increases the effectiveness of the massage. For example, if you have some experience with massage for back problems, you may consider supporting the stroking massage movements in between by using wands made of Aragonite, Aventurine, Serpentine, or Bloodstone. The back muscles will relax much faster and the effect will go much deeper. However, if you use a piece of Red Jasper or Basalt for such problems, it will take much longer for the relaxation effect to be noticeable.

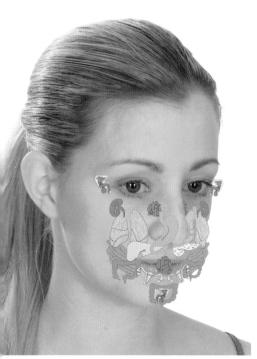

Reflexology Zones for Improving Blood Circulation in the Feet

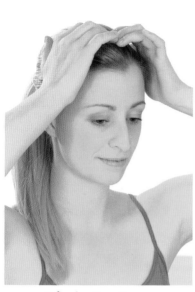

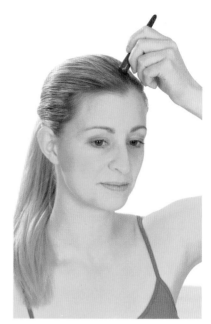

Reflexology Zone Massage
without Crystal Wands

Reflexology Zone Massage
with Mahogany Obsidian

Massaging with crystal wands has several immediate advantages. First of all, we are relieving the physical strain on ourselves by using crystal wands; we are being kinder to our hands, our most important tools. But the main reason for using crystal wands is this: the shape of the wand allows us to utilise the energetic quality of the crystal, thereby vastly increasing the efficacy

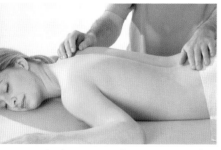

Back Massage with Serpentine Wand

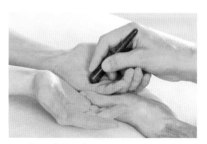

Crystal Wand: Energetic Instrument
and Relief for the Hands

and healing potential of the massage. It is, of course, important to choose the right crystal for the purpose, and this will be discussed in more detail in the next chapter. But, simply put, we will require crystals that provide us with three basic qualities: an activating, a balancing, and a neutral quality. Therefore, the basic set for massage with crystal wands includes three wands: Rock Crystal (neutral), Red Jasper (stimulating), and Aventurine (balancing) – see also the meaning of the crystals on pages 22-39.

These three basic qualities can then be amplified by fine-tuning with other crystal wands, and we have approximately 70 different crystal types at our disposal! However, questions can usually be reduced down to whether a treatment calls for stimulation or a calming effect, both of which can, of course, be carried out in many different ways.

No matter whether the goal is relaxation, composure, heightened awareness, or increased stamina, massaging with crystals brings about a perceptible and characteristic sense of wellbeing that underlies all other beneficial effects. The effects are long lasting, and if crystal wands are used in the treatment the desired state will be achieved more quickly and stabilized more permanently.

Last but certainly not least, in addition to enjoying the sheer beauty of crystal wands, we can employ these energetic tools in our everyday lives for self-massage, to help us feel good and to treat our own little niggles and complaints.

Crystal Wands Basic Set:
Rock Crystal, Red Jasper, Aventurine

Aesthetics and Form

One might think that aesthetics is not exactly the most important quality in a tool. Its form might suggest its function, obviously. However, the flow of energy within an object also depends on its form. In an energetic tool, the question of form becomes even more important due to the high energetic potential carried within its form and substance. When we perceive something as being

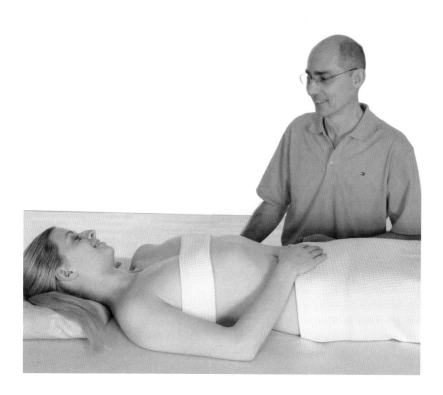

elegant or aesthetically pleasing, what we are experiencing is a 'felt sense' about the energetic flow within that object. We are familiar with this sensation from the shape or form of landscapes, rooms, or objects. If it is 'right', we feel good about it. A crystal wand possesses three qualities in its form that are energetically important, as well as being pleasant to the touch.

◎ First, there is the round, smooth, polished shape of the wand. Once we are holding one in our hands, it

is hard to put down. It is such a 'touchy-feely' object, we want to continuously move the crystal around in our hands, and we feel good doing it.

◎ The wand has no edges from which energy can escape sideways. The shape itself holds the energy inside the wand, so that its effectiveness is concentrated at the two ends. One end is round and allows us to use the crystal wand as we would a crystal sphere. This is especially useful for massage techniques that use flat movements, with applications where the aim is to distribute energy, or where an excess of energy needs to be conducted away. A different energetic state applies at the point, which runs into a rounded off tip. This is where energy is bundled. If this tip is used to concentrate on one point, zone or meridian, energy is conducted via that end of the crystal and the energetic state is intensified.

◎ When using either end, conducting energy away or conducting energy in, hold the crystal wand as you would a pencil or pen. This way the wand is easy to handle and can be used in a relaxed manner, without the therapist becoming tired.

Energy and Internal Communication

Now, for many people it is not enough to know that a method simply works. They want to know how and why. We now have the first scientific insights into the 'how' and 'why'. EEG measurements confirm the healing effect of crystals, as does a certified medical diagnostic device called the Biopulsar-Reflexograph, a biofeedback system created by a company called Auramed.*

As a result, we actually now have conclusive models for the efficacy of healing crystals.

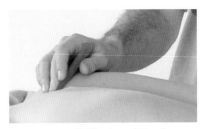

How to Hold a Crystal Wand

Quite apart from empirical evidence, we might ask ourselves, 'Why now?' 'Why, in the age of the computer and the Internet, have crystals emerged again for application in health and well-being?' Maybe because their effects can now, gradually, be explained? And maybe because we urgently require their assistance to meet the challenges of our times? Food for thought.

An explanation for the effects of crystals lies in their ability to conduct energies, to filter out individual qualities and to strengthen others.

◎ The most obvious energy forms are those that we can physically observe: lightning, thunder, electricity, or

* Friedrich Pelz, *Edelsteinfrequenz-Therapie* [Crystal Frequency Therapy], Spurbuchverlag, Baunach, 2004. For information on the Biopulsar-Reflexograph, see www.auramed.de

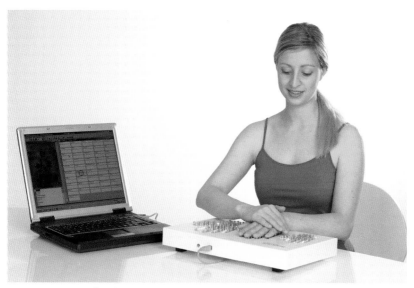

Reflexology Zone Massage with the Biopulsar-Reflexograph

the moving forces of engines, for example. We know too the power of sunlight, the Earth's gravity, the attraction of the Moon; and according to astrophysicists there are forces in the Universe the magnitude of which we can only dimly guess.

◎ Energies relating to crystals, however, only belong in part to these categories – they clearly go far beyond. The standard text on traditional Chinese medicine, the Nei Ching,* states that a human being swims like a fish in an ocean of energy, and its author was *not* referring, all those 2700 years ago, to the output of our high voltage electrical cables! He was referring to the energies radiated by all beings on Earth. Clairvoyant people in all cultures report that we possess life energy; it matters not whether we call it 'prana', 'chi', the 'aura' or 'breath'. Our technological achievements even allow us to depict these energies, and we can thus demonstrate that we are able to influence our surroundings beyond our physical boundaries.

* The *Nei Ching* has been ascribed to the legendary 'Yellow Emperor Huang Ti', who is believed to have lived around 2,700 BC. It was compiled during the 'age of the battling kingdoms' (221 BC – 220 AD).

Both physical energy and life energy play a role in the use of crystals. Both types of energy influence us, and can be filtered and amplified via crystals. It is a curious fact that we have long been utilizing the qualities of crystals in technology but still continue to question and doubt their effects on humans. What serious scientist would doubt the function of a ruby in laser technology, considering that we can bundle light with a ruby crystal and then use it to cut plates of steel like butter! And who nowadays would be able to manage without silicon crystals, with which we are able to pass on information? Crystals are the very basis of our computer chip technology! The filtering and amplifying functions of crystals for health and wellbeing are naturally a much subtler matter, but similarly powerful. We are able to influence moods and give the complex human organism impulses to help improve internal tuning.

So, what about side effects? And are there any restrictions on applications? Circumstances are similar to those in Homeopathy. From experience, the useful qualities of crystals unfold if the crystals' attributes are 'right' for the situation, and those that are not 'right' usually do not resonate. Only in about 10% of cases do the 'wrong' crystal wands cause unpleasant reactions. In the field of massage we can fortunately obtain immediate feedback and can therefore correct the choice of crystal wand if necessary. For this reason, always remain alert and maintain physical contact with the client; your stance should be relaxed, while at the same time retaining the courage to experiment. The positive effects will, as a rule, prevail strongly over any possible negative ones! This can be explained with the principle of resonance. If a maker of a bell strikes a tuning fork beside a bell and walks around the bell with it, the bell will at some point 'answer' and begin to resonate. This is the point at which it is in resonance with the note of the tuning fork. We are familiar with another phenomenon from professional singers like Enrico Caruso, or sopranos, who are able to shatter glass with certain notes they sing. Nowadays, resonances are even employed in the treatment of tinnitus;

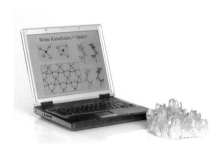

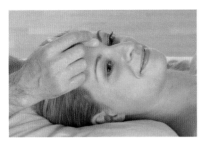

Resonance is the Basis of the Effect

'masking frequencies' are used to dampen the almost unbearable internal ringing noises in sufferers' ears.

Our organisms contain an orchestra of many voices consisting of vibrations and frequencies, for which research is only in its infancy. Besides the obvious 'rhythm sections' such as the pulse frequency and the rhythm of breathing, the cells also possess a 'working rhythm'. The highly organized formations, which we call our organs, can thus carry out their tasks optimally. This working frequency ensures good internal communication and internal tuning. Kidney cells have a different frequency to liver cells or the cells of the stomach. If an organ loses its proper rhythm, we will experience a restriction in its functioning, a feeling of dis-ease or illness. In addition, the organs also have to be tuned to each other. This task is mainly carried out by the autonomic nervous system, which penetrates and connects all the tissues of our bodies. In each and every one of us, this system has the unimaginable length of approximately 12 Earth circumferences, or, expressed in figures, about 480,000 kilometres. The best way to imagine this gigantic network is to liken it to the Internet, in which every organ possesses access terminals for sending and receiving e-mails.

Since the 1970s we have been familiar with an additional system in our internal communications systems. Research by Prof. Popp* has shown that all our cells are connected up by means of light communication. This means that, in addition to the 'solid network' of the autonomic nervous system, we also possess a light-based 'mobile function network' with which our cells are able to communicate with each other.

A further level of our internal tuning can be found in our energy body, the aura. This is where the 'ideas' or the 'basic concepts' of an organ have their roots. In connection with this we can refer back to traditional Chinese medicine and the ancient Indian Tantric chakra system. However, we too have our own access to these archetypal ideas about the organs. Who could doubt that

Fritz-Albert Popp, *Biophotonen – Neue Horizonte in der Medizin* [Bio-Photons – New Horizons in Medicine], (third edition), Hippokrates, Stuttgart, 2006

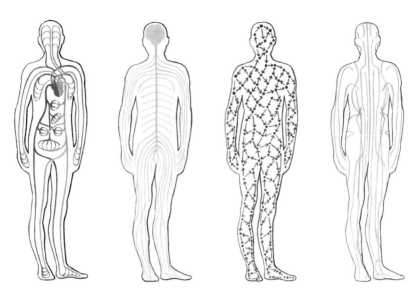

Communication within the Body and Internal Tuning
Blood circulation, Nervous System, Cell Communication, Meridian System

our hearts are connected with love? The archetype at work in the liver is a little more difficult to grasp, though it has been linked to the courage and determination of a warrior or an Amazon. The guardian function of the spleen can be better understood after a detailed observation of human anatomy. But all the organs resonate to a fundamental spiritual quality of energy. If this energy is properly balanced, we feel good; if it is not, then our spiritual life suffers both through our souls and through our bodies.

Archetypes are 'figures' within the human soul, and are known by all peoples worldwide. They describe fundamental psychic principles, which become effective through us. Moore and Gillette compared the functioning mechanisms of the archetypes to iron filings on a piece of paper, underneath which a magnet is passed back and forth. The visible movements of the iron filings represent perceptible psychic movements within us, while the magnet corresponds to the workings of the archetypal forces within our souls, which subconsciously steer our personalities. The influence of our organs on the way we feel and on our psyches really does allow us to surmise that there are hidden archetypal forces at work that have meaning in our lives.

We can influence these subtle energies with the use of the crystals, and by so doing can support and stabilize our internal communications. This goes a long way to explaining the healing power of crystals. Whether supporting autonomic toning through crystal massage, whether we aim to improve the light connections within our cells, or whether we wish to provide the fundamental ideas about our organs with new impulses, crystal wands provide us with a 'training staff' to help us raise our internal communications to top-level performance. The goal is to stabilize the body and the soul so that we are in the optimal position to master the challenges in our lives, and to preserve in us that which Hans-Georg Gadamer referred to as the 'pleasurable silence of the organs'.*

For practical application we have compiled a list of the 'training staffs'

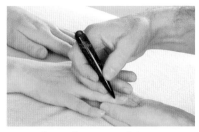

Crystals Regulate 'Internal Communications' through their Energetic Influence.

(the crystal wands), indicating which crystal wand is suited to which application, according to the qualities each crystal possesses. There is a wide range to choose from – about 70 different crystals are available as wands. However, we should always be aware that crystals are natural 'fruits of the Earth' and, as such, are not always unrestrictedly available. That said, you will always find suitable qualities among the crystals you can source; experience has shown that crystals find their way to us when we need them.

* Hans-Georg Gadamer, *The Enigma of Health: The Art of Healing in a Scientific Age*, Stanford University Press, 1996

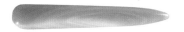

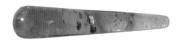

Agate brings about a pleasant feeling in the body, a gentle enveloping feeling within the skin. It is applied particularly for protection, safety, good sleep and better 'grounding'. Massage with Agate provides internal security and stability. On the physical side, Agate enhances the digestion, elimination, the tissue metabolism, the connective tissue and the skin. Agate enables and reinforces the ability to cope.
Energy quality: balancing
Availability: good

Amethyst lends inner peace and helps with sadness and grief. It is relaxing, but at the same time encourages an alert, conscious state. Massages with Amethyst before going to bed are reviving and help with understanding dreams. Amethyst has a calming effect and can therefore be very helpful after over exertion. Physically, a massage with Amethyst alleviates tension and headaches. Amethyst is good for the nerves and the skin, calms itching and sunburn, and lowers high blood pressure.
Energy quality: balancing
Availability: good

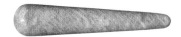

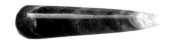

Amazonite is very helpful whenever too much stress leads to tension and pain. It is a wonderful healing crystal for joint complaints that arise from a variety of causes (overtaxing, strain, rheumatism, inflammation, liver problems, etc). In addition, Amazonite has a mood balancing effect, and is relaxing and pain relieving. It helps to calm the body.
Energy quality: balancing
Availability: low

Amethyst Quartz clears the head and encourages sobriety and alertness. It has a lifting effect on emotional lows, especially in cases of feelings of guilt and persistent grief. Amethyst Quartz also helps to dissolve 'blockages' and addictive behaviour. It enlivens in cases of persistent tiredness, but is also relaxing and pain relieving. Good for the lungs, nerves, and the skin; releases muscle tension, aids lazy digestion and constipation, and eases itching and sunburn.
Energy quality: balancing
Availability: good

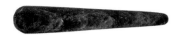

Apatite brings openness and sociability. It encourages liveliness, motivation and drive; helps with exhaustion; reduces irritability and aggression; and balances extreme alternating states of excessive activity and lack of drive. Physically, Apatite enhances growth, building up, and de-acidification. It promotes fitness, a healthy appetite, and mobilizes energy reserves; encourages the formation of cartilage, bone and teeth; and helps with posture problems, rickets, osteo-arthritis and joint complaints.
Energy quality: activating
Availability: rare

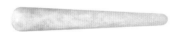

Aquamarine lends lightness and compo-sure, of a kind that is balanced with disci-pline and stamina. Physically it regulates growth and the hormone balance, and helps with allergies, especially hay fever. Aqua-marine is very good for tired and sore eyes – simply massage the area around the eyes with it. Applied regularly it also helps to reg-ulate squinting, short-sightedness or long-sightedness.
Energy quality: activating
Availability: rare

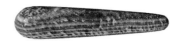

Aragonite stabilizes development (internal or external) that is happening too fast and causing instability, overtaxing or flagging interest. It lends flexibility, but also calms erratic feelings and behaviour. Aragonite calms in cases of oversensitivity and inner restlessness, and helps to bring about a feel-ing of being comfortable in the body. Physi-cally, Aragonite helps with liver and digestive complaints. It encourages harmonious growth, strengthens the muscles, and is helpful for problems of the spine, spinal discs, meniscus (cartilage in knee joint), and joints.
Energy quality: neutral
Availability: good

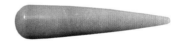

Aventurine (green) encourages relaxation and sleep. It helps switch off thoughts that go around and around in the head, as well as reducing stress, internal restlessness and nervousness. Green Aventurine is good for the skin when it is over-sensitive or irritated, and for heart complaints. It alleviates inflam-mations, sunburn and sunstroke, when applied in a very gentle, stroking massage. It can also be applied if lack of rest is leading to blockages of the body and/or mind.
Energy quality: balancing
Availability: good

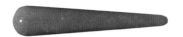

Aventurine (red) is a fortifying massage crystal. It lends composure and pragmatic drive; it also lends strength and internal security, activates and enlivens – but without over-stimulating. Physically, Red Aventurine stimulates the circulation, blood circulation, nerves and the senses. It strengthens the muscles and raises potency.
Energy quality: activating
Availability: rare

Basalt helps with being true to oneself and developing inner potential. It balances states of energetic fullness and lack, and is therefore activating and enlivening (a true 'power crystal'!), as well as relaxing and balancing. Basalt is wonderful for helping things flow. It encourages calmness and composure, but also an alert state of mind and quick reactions. Physically it promotes detoxification as well as encouraging digestion and elimination, which, in turn, supports the entire metabolic process.
Energy quality: activating
Availability: low

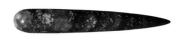

Bloodstone (Heliotrope) helps with setting boundaries so as to achieve a better grip on life. It alleviates irritability, aggressiveness and impatience, and revitalizes in cases of exhaustion and tiredness. Bloodstone is the 'echinacea' of crystals. It fortifies the immune system, which is why a massage with this crystal is very good for colds and the beginning stages of illness. Bloodstone also fortifies resistance to illness, relieves inflammation, detoxifies, relieves acidity, and also helps with heart complaints.
Energy quality: activating
Availability: low

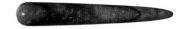

Blue Quartz is cooling and calming, bestows composure, and helps with nervousness. It encourages a calm and consistent approach to interesting and/or necessary undertakings. Blue Quartz lowers blood pressure and calms a fast pulse. It has a temperature-lowering effect, helps with chronic tension and alleviates pain. Blue Quartz may receive its colouring through a variety of inclusions (Azurite, Dumortierite, rutiles, and Tourmaline); however, the qualities described apply to all Blue Quartzes.
Energy quality: balancing
Availability: low

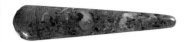

Brecciated Jasper has a building-up and enlivening effect. It helps in dealing with crises, and recovering after a defeat. Brecciated Jasper encourages a readiness to meet conflicts, and helps with overcoming difficulties. Physically it has a vitalizing effect and helps in cases of weakness and tiredness, and stimulates the circulation. It also supports self-healing, and promotes the protective functions of the entire organism.
Energy quality: activating
Availability: good

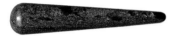

Bronzite is like a 'pocket island' in times of great stress and challenge. It lends the necessary drive, but also brings inner peace and recovery in times of exhaustion. Bronzite helps retain a clear head and a sense of control during times of persistent stress. Physically, Bronzite alleviates pain and dissolves tension and cramps. It fortifies the nerves, muscles and bones, and eases digestive complaints stemming from nervous stress.
Energy quality: activating
Availability: low

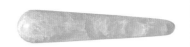

Calcite (blue) has a calming effect, and engenders internal stability and security. It supports the ability to discriminate, and helps when activities are being carried out with more effort than is actually needed. Physically it is very good for the lymphatic system, mucous membranes, skin, the large intestines, connective tissue, bones and teeth. For treating teeth, use it to massage externally along the jaw. Blue Calcite is also suitable for massaging children who are suffering from growing pains.
Energy quality: balancing
Availability: rare

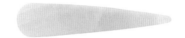

Calcite (orange) is a sunny, fortifying crystal that lends a very good feeling to the body and strengthens acceptance of oneself. During massage it lends a pleasurable inner warmth, which strengthens one's confidence and trust. Orange Calcite firms up the tissues, makes the muscles pliable and strengthens the bones. It has a very good effect on the entire belly and gut system, as well as on the digestion, the connective tissue, skin, joints and bones.
Energy quality: activating
Availability: good

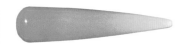

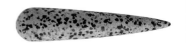

Carnelian* makes a person open and sociable. It has an activating, enlivening effect, helps us approach others, and brings drive, courage and good humour. Carnelian provides support in overcoming difficulties when working towards a goal. Physically, it stimulates the small intestine, the metabolism, the cardiovascular system and the blood circulation. It also promotes the absorption of vitamins, nutrients and minerals, as well as improving the fluid qualities of the blood.

Energy quality: activating
Availability: low

Dalmatian Jasper (Aplite) has a strengthening, building up, and emotionally balancing effect. It stimulates the clear and careful thinking-through of a project, with reflection at each step along the way, and then the active realisation of the goal. Dalmatian Jasper also improves body perception, and especially makes physical perceptions much clearer. As a crystal used for massage, it supports balanced firmness and flexibility, as well as stable nerves and a good ability to react.

Energy quality: neutral
Availability: good

Chalcedony (as a blue-banded crystal) enables free flow whenever we feel inhibited or feel that obstacles are preventing us from doing what we want. It makes us open, communicative and 'on the ball'. Physically, massage with this crystal encourages the flow of body fluids, especially the lymph. The functions of the glands, kidneys and bladder are also supported. Blue-banded Chalcedony has a cooling and calming effect, which may also enable it to lower a high temperature or high blood pressure.

Energy quality: neutral
Availability: low

Dolomite encourages self-realisation and the development of abilities. It lends a sense of stability, patience, and satisfaction with oneself. Dolomite alleviates stress and improves sleep. Physically, it helps with 'muscular hangovers', cramp and tension, as well as the associated effects on the internal organs. Dolomite regulates the metabolism, muscle tone, blood pressure, and blood circulation through the tissues. It can also be employed for joint complaints and posture problems.

Energy quality: activating
Availability: low

---

* Usually, carnelians that are worked into wands are treated at high temperatures to make their orangey red colour more 'attractive'. Whether or how much this heating technique changes the effects of Carnelian is not yet known.

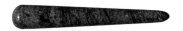

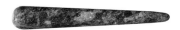

Dumortierite lends composure and ease (the 'take-it-easy crystal'). It has a cooling, calming, relaxing effect and eases anxieties, depression, nervousness, internal restlessness and stress. Dumortierite helps us to 'get a grip' on life and thus reduces worries, compulsions and internal tension. As a crystal used for massage, it is helpful with pain, cramp, headaches and travel sickness, even with nausea and vomiting.
Energy quality: balancing
Availability: good

Epidote (Unakite) is a very good crystal for treating exhaustion, after physical over-exertion, as well as after a long illness or a period of mental stress. On the soul level, Epidote (Unakite) helps to overcome frustration stemming from a sense of failure. It strengthens the gall bladder, the liver and the kidneys, supports regenerative abilities, and accelerates the healing processes. In massage, Epidote (Unakite) has a very good building up and strengthening effect.
Energy quality: activating
Availability: good

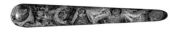

Eldarite (Kabamba) encourages vitality, bestows inner strength, and protects one against external pressure, anxiety, negativity and foreign influences. It strengthens the immune system, helps with severe infections, and encourages regeneration after illness. In addition, Eldarite (Kabamba) is very good for the skin. It opens the pores, supports perspiration and thus detoxification. A very good massage crystal for the sauna or before detox-baths.
Energy quality: activating
Availability: good

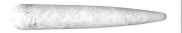

Feldspar, white (Plagioclase) improves perception and the ability to feel. It encourages attentiveness and sensitivity to our surroundings, and helps us to observe old familiar things from a new perspective. Physically, white Feldspar supports the pliability of the muscles and the flexibility of the tissues. It loosens feelings of tightness in the chest area, makes breathing easier, and relieves intestinal complaints and skin diseases.
Energy quality: neutral
Availability: rare

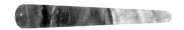

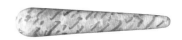

Fluorite increases physical and mental flexibility. It brings structure and order into life and helps with disorders relating to stress, learning, and concentration. Fluorite clears the head, dissolves energetic blockages, alleviates chronic tension and helps with posture problems. Fluorite stimulates the nerves; is good for the skin, tissues, bones, cartilage and joints; and helps with coughs and hoarseness, as well as with irritated or diseased mucous membranes.
Energy quality: neutral
Availability: low (fragile!)

Graphic Granite is fortifying, strengthening and enlivening, and helps us to better manage our own energies and resources. It improves boundary perception and encourages us to care for ourselves, and therefore improves our resiliency and makes us better able to deal with stressful situations. In massage, Graphic Granite helps with back problems, especially those associated with psychological burdens, lack of grounding and physical weakness.
Energy quality: neutral
Availability: good

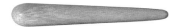

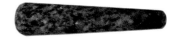

Fossil Wood gives us an all-round good feeling about our bodies and being on this Earth. It helps us compose ourselves, strengthens us, helps us to 'be' in the body, and accept ourselves as we are. All these things improve our relationship with our own bodies. Fossil Wood relaxes and strengthens, fortifies the digestion, promotes detoxification and elimination, and helps with excess weight when it is due to a lack of grounding. In addition, it has a warming effect, especially for those cold extremities.
Energy quality: balancing
Availability: good

Granite (blue) connects new insights with old experiences. It lends strength and composure, especially when seeking form and structure in a new phase of life. Use it to gather strength from a peaceful state. Blue Granite firms up new ideas so that they can take shape and be realized. Physically, it helps balance coldness and warmth. This, in turn, stabilizes the circulation and promotes a more balanced muscle tone.
Energy quality: activating
Availability: low

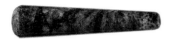

Granite (brown) brings stability, strength and good grounding. It strengthens and stabilizes during difficult and stressful times, encourages staying power, and helps the step-by-step realisation of ideas and goals. Brown Granite helps with weakness and tiredness, has a warming effect, and stimulates the digestion, metabolism and circulation. Brown Granite strengthens the muscles, tendons and ligaments and thus helps us remain 'upright'.

Energy quality: activating
Availability: good

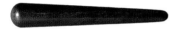

Hematite lends power and vitality. It strengthens the will, brings unfulfilled wishes to light, and stimulates us to improve our own life circumstances. Hematite fortifies endurance during challenging work or other demanding circumstances. Physically, it supports the formation of blood and the transportation of oxygen within the body, thereby increasing vitality. Massages with Hematite vitalize, improve blood circulation and are warming; they make us alert and ready for action.

Energy quality: activating
Availability: good

Iron Quartz makes us alert, aware and attentive. It sharpens the senses and helps process impressions quickly. Physically, Iron Quartz has a pleasantly enlivening effect; it fortifies the autonomic nervous system and thus improves the harmonious interplay of the organs. Iron Quartz cleanses and strengthens the connective tissue and fortifies and rejuvenates the skin.

Energy quality: activating
Availability: low

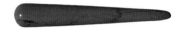

Jasper (red) is the crystal for activity and dynamism. It enhances courage and the ability to assert oneself, lends energy and drive, and helps with persistent weakness and tiredness. Physically, red Jasper stimulates the circulation, thus having a warming effect if one is susceptible to feeling cold. Massages with red Jasper are perceived to be strongly activating, so they should not be carried out late in the evening. Red Jasper is very good for boosting energy levels that are low due to difficult matters arising in life.

Energy quality: activating
Availability: good

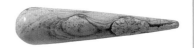

Labradorite has a cooling effect if a person is too hot, and a warming effect if they are too cold. It fortifies the intuition, deepens the feeling nature, and supports mediumistic abilities. Labradorite helps with understanding of the roots or reasons for illnesses and to find solutions for conflicts and problems. Physically, it frees the tissues of toxins and toxic deposits, and thereby also helps with rheumatism and gout. Labradorite has a calming, blood-pressure-lowering effect.
Energy quality: neutral
Availability: low

Landscape Jasper lends stamina and quiet steadfastness. It strengthens us in situations of longstanding stress and, after failures, helps us continue making new attempts at success. Physically, Landscape Jasper supports digestion and elimination (stomach, pancreas and intestines). It fortifies the spleen and the cleansing of the connective tissue and in that way also helps with food sensitivities and other allergies, hay fever for example.
Energy quality: activating
Availability: good

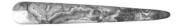

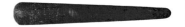

Lace Agate (Agate in the form of filigree) is very good for supplying energy to, and eliminating energy from, connective tissue. It stimulates the metabolism and fortifies the blood vessels and the intestines, and is therefore very good for varicose veins and haemorrhoids. Lace Agate lends dexterity, flexibility and dynamism, as well as mental flexibility.
Energy quality: activating
Availability: low

Lapis Lazuli with Pyrite* brings openness, self-confidence and self-awareness. It helps us find 'space' when we feels restricted, and makes the body calm but ready to react. Lapis Lazuli with Pyrite helps us to communicate with others and express our needs, and by so doing we gain a sense of control over life. It is good for throat problems of all kinds, purifies the blood, strengthens the nerves, and is generally vitalizing.

Please note, Lapis Lazuli massages may slow the menstrual cycle.
Energy quality: activating (with Pyrite); balancing (without Pyrite)
Availability: low

---

* Many of the effects listed here are generally applicable to Lapis Lazuli and are independent of the Pyrite content. The main difference with the presence of Pyrite is the experiencing of things in an intensely extroverted

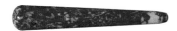

Lapis Lazuli without Pyrite* brings honesty and genuineness. It helps a person be who they truly are. At the same time, it also encourages sociability and helps support and maintain friendships. Lapis Lazuli without Pyrite fortifies a sense of responsibility for oneself and improves discernment and intelligence. It may also help bring about the feeling of being comfortable in the body. Lapis Lazuli without Pyrite regulates the functioning of the thyroid gland, has a cooling effect, is calming, and lowers blood pressure. Massages with Lapis Lazuli may also slow down the menstrual cycle.
Energy quality: balancing
Availability: low

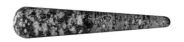

Leopardstone Jasper (Rhyolite) bestows firmness and stability, but at the same time, flexibility and adaptability. It brings about a balance between activity and rest, and improves sleep. Leopardstone Jasper makes clear that which needs doing in life and provides the stimulation necessary to do it. Physically, it stimulates digestion and elimination and helps with skin complaints and hardened tissue. Massages with Leopardstone Jasper have an 'after effect', meaning that the effect often comes a little while after the treatment. This is especially true of its loosening effect on hardened tissue.
Energy quality: activating
Availability: low

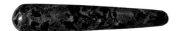

Larvikite (Syenite) helps with working through complicated sets of circumstances and understanding them. It has a calming effect in cases of violent emotions and encourages sobriety and neutrality, which, in turn, has a physically calming effect on the nerves and the brain. Larvikite encourages detoxification of the tissues, has a cooling effect and lowers blood pressure. As a massage crystal it has a desensitizing effect on highly sensitive people.
Energy quality: neutral
Availability: rare

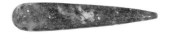

Lepidolite protects and helps in the creation of proper boundaries, allowing rest, relaxation and inner peace. It helps to ward off influences from without and helps us concentrate on the essential things. Physically it alleviates joint and nerve pain, pain arising from the ischium, and neuralgic pain. Lepidolite also strengthens and protects the skin. It soothes itching and helps with skin complaints.
Energy quality: balancing
Availability: low

way, with greater impulsiveness, a stronger means of expression, and especially the raising of blood pressure! Without Pyrite, however, Lapis Lazuli lowers blood pressure.

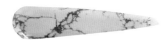

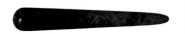

Magnesite has a deeply relaxing effect, and helps with cramps and various kinds of pain. Massages with Magnesite improve patience and ease irritability and fearfulness. Physically, Magnesite is a blessing for the muscles and the connective tissue. Magnesite helps with headaches, migraines, 'muscular hangovers', stomach complaints, nausea, back complaints and joint pains. It can also be applied supportively in detox programs. Magnesite acts as a preventive for deposits in the blood vessels and for heart attacks.
Energy quality: balancing
Availability: good

Mahogany Obsidian lends power, initiative and renewed drive. It dissolves upsets caused by insults, put-downs and unjustified accusations. It has an enlivening effect and brings about spontaneous motivation. A massage with Mahogany Obsidian physically stimulates blood circulation and brings inner warmth, particularly for those that have a tendency to feel cold and have cold hands and feet. In addition, Mahogany Obsidian stimulates the metabolism and encourages wound healing.
Energy quality: activating
Availability: good

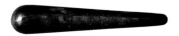

Magnetite brings a sense of orientation, and hones the ability to react. It stimulates us to follow higher ideals and helps us distinguish between useful and useless things. Magnetite is very strongly activating (therefore contraindications include nervousness, inner restlessness, hyperactivity and similar!). It stimulates the flow of energy, the functions of the glands, the liver, and the production of gall. Used in massage, Magnetite has a nerve stimulating effect, which is why it may help with weakness, paralysis and numbness.
Energy quality: activating
Availability: rare

Marble supports changes in existing life circumstances and lends the courage, strength and renewed energy to change seemingly irresolvable situations. It helps to free us from dissatisfaction on the soul level, and opens us to new perspectives. Marble encourages development in children, as well as the bodily processes involved in strengthening and renewing. It alleviates allergies, stimulates detoxification and elimination processes, and strengthens the spleen, kidneys, intestines, tissues and skin.
Energy quality: neutral
Availability: good

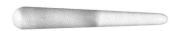

Mookaite brings liveliness, alertness, flexibility, and promotes interest in life. It encourages variety, fun, and the wish for intense experiences. Mookaite helps maintain a balance between external activities and the digestion of impressions arising from those activities. Massages with Mookaite bring a pleasurable body feeling as it has both a relaxing and gently enlivening effect. Mookaite makes us soft and strong, encourages cleansing of the blood and wound healing, and strengthens the spleen, the liver and the immune system.
Energy quality: activating
Availability: good

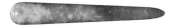

Moss Agate dissolves internal tension and has a liberating effect when there is a feeling of heaviness, depression or restriction. It brings relief to the soul, helps loosen deep-seated anxieties, and encourages hope and trust. Moss Agate boosts awareness, loosens blocked communication and encourages a lively intellect. Physically, Moss Agate has an immune-strengthening effect, lowers a high temperature, and soothes inflammation. It stimulates lymph flow and the cleansing of the tissues, mucous membranes and the respiratory tract.
Energy quality: neutral
Availability: good

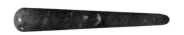

Nephrite brings inner balance, and a balance between activity and rest. It alleviates impatience and aggression, helps reduce tension and grief, and renders us insusceptible to external pressure. Nephrite helps with indecisiveness, making us creative and happy to act. It strengthens the kidneys, thus bringing more vitality, and encourages detoxification. Through massage, it is good for treating tinnitus and migraine.
Energy quality: neutral
Availability: good

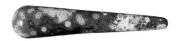

Ocean Jasper lends the courage to face life and brings hope. It has a mood-lifting effect and motivates, making us able to meet demands while at the same time relaxing us and encouraging refreshing sleep. Ocean Jasper is very suitable for massages intended for fortifying the person, especially when new energy is required to meet challenging times, or after illness. Physically, it firms up the tissues. It stimulates the lymph flow, detoxification processes and the immune system; it alleviates inflammation, and inhibits the growth of cysts and tumours.
Energy quality: neutral
Availability: low

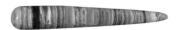

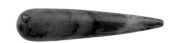

Onyx Marble (Aragonite Calcite Rock) brings internal relief when confronted with persistent demands. It makes us calmer and more relaxed, freer and more sensitive, encouraging the development of the soul and the body as well as supporting all rhythmic life processes. In massage Onyx Marble it is at once calming and fortifying, and is helpful for complaints related to the spine, the spinal discs, the knee joint, and the joints in general. It fortifies the liver and harmonizes growth.
Energy quality: neutral
Availability: good

Prase Quartz fosters gentleness, calms heated feelings, and makes it easier to resolve conflicts. It encourages conscious control; even when violent emotions rage, it helps us keep our actions in check. Prase Quartz helps with bladder problems; alleviates pain, bruising and swelling; has a cooling and fever-lowering effect; and helps with the influence of radiation, such as sunburn and sunstroke (gently stroke the affected area!).
Energy quality: balancing
Availability: low

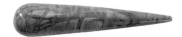

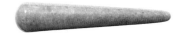

Picasso Marble (limestone) makes us temperate and reality-based. It helps us stand firmly on the ground, regard the facts, objectively define problems and then solve them. Picasso Marble helps us stay true to the Self, to recognize what is essential, and lends the necessary persistence to carry ideas through to realisation. It detoxifies and firms up the connective tissue, helps reduce water retention, strengthens the bones and supports intestinal activity.
Energy quality: neutral
Availability: good

Rhodonite is a wound healer both on the physical and soul level. It helps us to forgive, encourages mutual understanding and firms up friendships. It is physically very good for rubbing into scarred tissue, helping it to become more pliable and encouraging regeneration. It is very good for the muscles, connective tissue and the circulation. It strengthens the heart, encourages fertility, and helps with diseases of the immune system.
Energy quality: activating
Availability: low

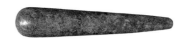

Rock Crystal, being a neutral, clear quartz crystal, is practically universally applicable. It lends energy in the right amounts and encourages clarity. Massages with Rock Crystal are very satisfying and relaxing, but at the same time bring renewed vitality. Rock Crystal is cooling and refreshing, alleviates pain, increases awareness, opens up the senses, and encourages a willingness to take in new things. Because Rock Crystal has fortifying qualities, it can help one perceive the physical body more consciously.
Energy quality: neutral
Availability: good

Ruby in Disthene lends determination and drive, and boosts willpower and self-realisation. It engenders consistency, helps with overcoming crises, and preserves the joie de vivre, even in difficult situations. In massage, it helps us emerge from absolute energy low points, and mobilizes the spirit and life force. It is very good for nervous complaints, circulatory problems, heart rhythm irregularities, and a tight feeling in the chest.
Energy quality: activating
Availability: rare

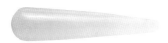

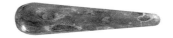

Rose Quartz is beautiful for harmonious and loving treatments. It makes us sensitive and empathetic, and encourages genuineness, helpfulness, and compassion. Rose Quartz brings us to an awareness of our needs, and therefore sometimes encourages relaxation and sometimes stimulation. It improves the 'feeling' of one's body, is good for the heart, and encourages the entire blood circulation through the tissues, which leads to a healthy, rosy skin colour. Rose Quartz encourages fertility and helps with sexual difficulties.
Energy quality: neutral
Availability: good

Ruby in Fuchsite has a tension-alleviating effect in cases of stress and extreme strain. It encourages composure and self-determination, lends good sleep, and envelops us in a feeling of secure protection. Ruby Fuchsite supports responsibility for the Self and helps us to cope with our own problems. Physically, Ruby Fuchsite has a pain-alleviating effect, and is very helpful with paralysis, rheumatism, inflammation and skin diseases, as well as heart and back problems.
Energy quality: neutral
Availability: low

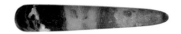

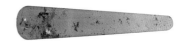

Sardonyx lends friendliness, helpfulness and inner balance. It intensifies perception, encourages the working of all the organs of the senses (nose, ears, mouth, etc.), and helps with tinnitus. Sardonyx strengthens the spleen and the immune system, has a supportive effect on the blood circulatory system, gently detoxifies, and encourages lymph flow. It is therefore very helpful for rebalancing the entire 'system' after an illness. Sardonyx also helps with influenza and colds, especially the associated joint pain.
Energy quality: activating
Availability: low

Smoky Quartz* is the classic anti-stress crystal. It allows internal tension to flow away, heightens the ability to bear burdens, and helps us not to 'allow ourselves' to become stressed. Physically, too, it eases back problems and tight jaw muscles. Smoky Quartz is generally pain-relieving, strengthens the nerves, and helps to compensate for the effects of radiation.
Energy quality: balancing
Availability: rare

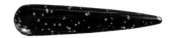

Scolesite encourages team spirit. It helps with weakness of the will and drive, stems the draining of energy through excessive activity, cools sexual urges, and brings beneficial sleep. Scolesite allows life energy to flow properly, makes us fit and productive, and strengthens the body's constitution. It sharpens hearing and regenerates exhausted kidney energy, and helps with complaints involving the bones, ears and kidneys. Scolesite encourages fertility in men and women.
Energy quality: neutral
Availability: rare

Snowflake Obsidian helps with pain, psychological and physical blockages, and the consequences of accidents, injuries and operations. It dissolves states of shock, even shocks on the cellular level, and thereby helps to overcome blockages in healing. Massage with Snowflake Obsidian helps with irregularities in blood circulation, cold extremities, as well as general fatigue, weakness and lack of motivation. Snowflake Obsidian raises energy on all levels.
Energy quality: activating
Availability: low

---

* In order to create Smoky Quartz from colourless crystals, Quartz is sometimes irradiated with radioactive substances. Unfortunately, that turns the effect into the opposite, and these Quartzes then react more in a tension-heightening manner. As irradiation with gemological methods can often not be detected, please pay close attention to the effects on and reactions of your client when using Smoky Quartz.

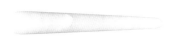

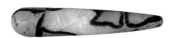

Snow Quartz encourages attentiveness and helps us to recognize our own potential and to live fully. It enlivens, energizes, and alleviates blockages to the breathing caused by tension and stress. Snow Quartz calms inner restlessness and quickly and easily alleviates pain. It helps with spinal and joint complaints, as well as with weakness and feelings of numbness in the extremities. Snow Quartz cleanses and firms up the skin, has a stimulating effect on the lymph system and stimulates the circulation.

Energy quality: neutral
Availability: good

Septarian helps us to establish proper boundaries while still remaining open. It helps us remain steadfast but without closing off, especially in difficult situations. Septarian is part Calcite (activating) and part Clay (balancing). It has a building up and strengthening effect (Calcite), and encourages de-acidification, detoxification and elimination (Clay). In massage, it dissolves hardening, growths and tumours in tissues. Septarian also helps with intestinal and skin complaints, especially those due to over-acidification.

Energy quality: neutral (Calcite part is activating; Clay part is balancing)
Availability: rare

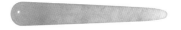

Selenite lends firmness, shields against outside influences, calms us when we feel irritated and hyperactive (especially when at the point of 'losing it'), and helps us retreat to find peace and rest. It firms up the tissues and has a pain-relieving effect, especially with the consequences of over-exertion. In massage, it can also be used for dissolving muscle hardening.

Energy quality: neutral
Availability: good (not as a wand, but in similar forms)

Serpentine* has a strongly relaxing effect and helps with nervousness, restlessness, mood swings and a feeling of lack of protection. Serpentine makes it possible to form proper personal boundaries, and to maintain inner peace. Massages with Serpentine may dissolve sexual blockages, especially if inner tension is causing an inability to achieve orgasm. Physically, Serpentine helps with heart rhythm irregularities, and with kidney, stomach and menstrual complaints.

Energy quality: balancing
Availability: good

* Serpentine is available in a transparent variety (known as China Jade); it can also be yellowish green with dark dots (Chytha), or it can be dark green with silvery stripes (Silver Eye).

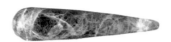 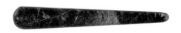

Sodalite helps create free space and time for the things we really want to experience in life. It supports us in remaining true to ourselves, helps us to consciously change behaviour patterns, and encourages consistent self-development. Massage with Sodalite has a cooling effect, calms heat sensitivity, lowers fevers and blood pressure, and helps with inflammation of the throat and hoarseness. Sodalite supports the water balance in the body and alleviates dryness of the eyes, skin, mucous membranes, etc.

Energy quality: balancing
Availability: good

Stichtite in Serpentine helps with turbulent moods, lends inner peace and emotional openness, encourages relaxation and the dissolving of muscle cramps, and helps with over-acidification, heartburn and stomach complaints. It improves the pliability of muscles, connective tissue and the skin, and alleviates inflammation and rheumatic complaints. Stichtite in Serpentine is a very strong pain-relieving crystal.

Energy quality: balancing
Availability: rare

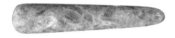 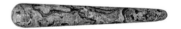

Sunstone promotes optimism and the enjoyment of life. It encourages self-acceptance, lends joie de vivre, and stimulates us to see the positive sides of life. Sunstone has a mood lifting, anti-depressant effect and helps with anxieties and worries. Physically, it harmonizes the autonomic nervous system and thus improves the quality of the blood and stabilizes the circulation.

Energy quality: activating
Availability: rare

Stromatolite helps with working through accumulated experiences, and thereby promotes growth. It also strengthens us in the ability to adapt and to remain flexible, while also remaining firm with our point of view. Stromatolite is very good for the digestion and eases tension in the belly (and eases worries too!). It encourages the proper working of the metabolism, supports detoxification and elimination, improves the intestinal flora, and helps with a lazy intestine. As a massage crystal it dissolves tensions and cramps, and reinforces the connective tissue and the skin.

Energy quality: balancing
Availability: good

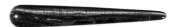

Tiger's Eye lends peace when everything is 'going haywire'. It helps us to compose ourselves and to recognize what's what, and allows some distance from the impressions that rush in from outside ourselves. Tiger's Eye helps us navigate through difficult phases of life without losing courage. It therefore also alleviates the physical consequences of stress. It calms overwrought nerves, stops the excessive production of adrenaline and other stress hormones, alleviates pain, and helps us return home to ourselves.
Energy quality: activating
Availability: good

Tourmaline Schorl (Black Tourmaline) is an important protective crystal. It helps us find composure and neutrality, reduces our internal tension, and helps us become energetically 'transfluent' so that nothing can attach itself to us. Thus it protects us from the influence of electro-smog, and even energetic and psychic attacks. Schorl is very good for the energy flow of the nerves and the meridians. It creates internal energy balancing, alleviates pain and tension, and helps with motor problems, feelings of numbness, and paralysis. Massaging with Schorl is also helpful for the energetic unblocking of scars.
Energy quality: neutral
Availability: rare

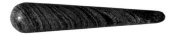

Tiger Iron mobilizes that 'tiger in the tank', lending force, dynamism, strength and masses of energy. It provides new impulses when there has been a longing for change. Physically, Tiger Iron stimulates blood formation, the circulation, and the blood circulation. It brings oxygen into all the cells, helps with severe exhaustion, increases vitality, and makes tired people feel lively again. Caution: Tiger Iron massages in the evening can be so stimulating that a client might not be able sleep afterwards.
Energy quality: activating
Availability: low

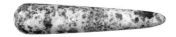

Tree Agate encourages inner peace and protection. It lends persistence and stability, and instils courage in situations where there is a feeling of powerlessness and vulnerability. Tree Agate helps us stand firm in the face of challenges. Physically it ensures vitality, stable health and a strong immune system. It improves resistance to frequent infection.
Energy quality: neutral
Availability: low

Overview of Energy Qualities

Activating Crystal Wands	**Neutral Crystal Wands**	**Balancing Crystal Wands**
Lace Agate	Aragonite	Agate
Apatite	Chalcedony, blue-banded	Amazonite
Aquamarine	Dalmatian Jasper (Aplite)	Amethyst
Aventurine, red	Feldspar (white)	Amethyst Quartz
Basalt	Fluorite	Aventurine, green
Bloodstone (Heliotrope)	Labradorite	Blue Quartz
Brecciated Jasper	Larvikite (Syenite)	Calcite, blue
Bronzite	Marble	Dumortierite
Carnelian	Moss Agate	Fossil Wood.
Calcite, orange	Nephrite	Lapis Lazuli without Pyrite
Dolomite	Ocean Jasper	Lepidolite
Eldarite (Kabamba)	Picasso Marble (Lime-	Magnesite
Epidote (Unakite)	stone)	Prase Quartz
Granite	Onyx Marble (Aragonite	Serpentine
Hematite	Calcite rock)	Smoky Quartz
Iron Quartz	Rock Crystal	Sodalite
Jasper, red	Rose Quartz	Stichtite in Serpentine
Landscape Jasper	Ruby in Fuchsite	Stromatolite
Lapis Lazuli with Pyrite	Graphic Granite	
Leopardstone Jasper	Scolesite	
(Rhyolite)	Selenite	
Magnesite	Septarian	
Mahagony Obsidian	Snow Quartz	
Mookaite	Tourmaline Schorl.	
Rhodonite	Tree Agate	
Ruby in Disthene		
Sardonyx		
Snowflake Obsidian		
Sunstone		
Tiger's Eye		
Tiger Iron		

Overview of range of applications

3 = especially applicable

2 = can easily be applied in this area

1 = this aspect is a 'side effect'

– = not suitable or negligible for this application

	Wellness	Beauty	Power	Relaxation	Protection
Agate	1	2	-	2	3
Agate, Lace Agate	3	2	2	-	1
Amazonite	1	1	-	3	1
Amethyst Quarz	2	3	1	2	3
Amethyst	1	3	1	3	2
Apatite	2	-	3	-	1
Aquamarine	1	2	2	1	1
Aragonite, brown	3	2	1	1	2
Aventurine, green	2	1	-	3	1
Aventurine, red	2	3	3	-	-
Basalt	2	1	3	1	2
Bloodstone (Heliotrope)	3	1	2	1	3
Blue Quartz	2	3	-	3	1
Brecciated Jasper	1	1	3	-	3
Bronzite	3	1	3	3	2
Calcite, blue	3	2	1	3	2
Calcite, orange	3	2	3	-	1
Carnelian	2	3	3	-	1
Chalcedony	3	3	1	2	2
Dalmatian Jasper (Aplite)	1	1	3	-	2
Dolomite	2	3	2	-	1
Dumortierite	3	3	1	2	2
Eldarite (Kabamba)	3	2	1	-	3
Epidote (Unakite)	2	1	3	-	1
Feldspar, white	3	2	1	1	2
Fluorite	2	3	1	1	2
Fossil Wood	3	1	2	2	2
Granite (all varieties)	2	1	3	-	1
Graphic Granite (Hebrew Stone)	2	1	3	1	2
Hematite	2	1	3	-	1
Iron Quartz	2	2	3	-	2
Jasper, red	1	1	3	-	3
Labradorite	3	3	1	1	2

	Wellness	Beauty	Power	Relaxation	Protection
Landscape Jasper	2	1	3	1	1
Lapis Lazuli with Pyrite	1	2	3	1	3
Lapis Lazuli without Pyrite	1	2	1	3	2
Larvikite (Syenite)	2	1	-	3	1
Lepidolite	2	3	-	3	3
Magnesite	3	2	-	3	1
Magnetite	-	-	3	-	2
Mahagony Obsidian	2	2	3	-	2
Marble	3	2	2	2	3
Mookaite	3	3	2	1	2
Moss Agate	2	2	1	2	3
Nephrite	3	3	2	2	3
Ocean Jasper	2	2	2	1	3
Onyx Marble (Aragonite Calcite)	3	2	1	1	2
Picasso Marble (Limestone)	1	1	3	-	1
Prase Quartz	2	1	-	3	1
Rhodonite	2	3	3	1	2
Rhyolite	2	-	2	1	-
Rock Crystal	3	3	2	1	2
Rose Quartz	3	3	2	2	2
Ruby in Disthene	2	2	3	1	3
Ruby in Fuchsite	2	2	2	2	3
Sardonyx	2	3	2	2	2
Scolesite	3	2	3	2	3
Selenite	2	3	-	3	3
Septarian	2	2	2	2	3
Serpentine (all varieties)	2	3	-	3	3
Smoky Quartz	3	3	2	2	2
Snow Quartz	2	3	2	1	2
Snowflake Obsidian	2	1	3	-	3
Sodalite	2	2	1	3	2
Stichtite in Serpentine	3	3	1	3	3
Stromatolite	2	3	1	2	2
Sunstone	3	3	3	2	2
Tiger Iron	1	-	3	-	3
Tiger's Eye	2	2	2	1	3
Tourmaline, black (Schorl)	2	2	2	3	3
Tree Agate	3	1	2	1	1

Handling

Unfortunately, crystals are not as eternal and permanent as we might imagine. There are some very robust types, such as Agate, Jasper and Nephrite, but most of them are quite delicate and easily broken, especially when in the slim shape of wands. Most delicate of them all is Fluorite, in which 'split layers' are often clearly visible. Split layers can suddenly become split-off points if we knock the wand against a hard object or drop it. Careful use of crystal wands is therefore really important. For professional masseurs we even recommend keeping two of each of the most important and most used crystals.

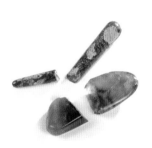

Energetic influences can also lead to crystal wands splitting along their hidden cracks. If a crystal takes on too much energetic load during a treatment session, its crystal lattice will become stressed. Hitherto invisible cracks may open up, leading to clouding or even to the wand breaking completely. Colours may also fade or change; in the case of Snowflake Obsidian, the 'flakes' consisting of Feldspar crystals may even grow out of the dark Obsidian matrix. These changes, as a rule, will not reduce the effect of the wand, except if the colours completely disappear or the crystal actually breaks. In order to reduce this risk, crystal wands should be regularly cleansed.

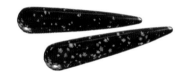

Cleansing and Care

Before first use, as well as regularly after every massage, you should thoroughly cleanse your crystals.

If you have worked with massage oils, first remove the remains of the oil and rub the crystals dry properly. If necessary, you may also disinfect the wands with alcohol.

Afterwards, they should be thoroughly cleansed of the energies and information they have absorbed.

For this, hold your crystal wand for a minute or longer under running water

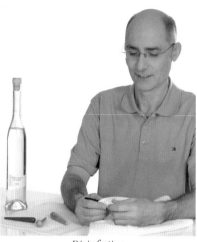

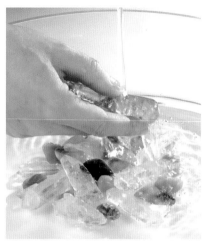

Disinfection

Cleansing on the Energetic Level under Running Water

and rub it hard with your fingers. You will discover that the surface of the wand, which initially might have felt a little 'soapy', will create more resistance after a while, so that the fingers no longer glide so easily across it. This shows that the absorbed charges have been removed.

Then remove the crystals from the water and lay them on an Amethyst druse or Amethyst druse piece. Amethyst liberates the crystals from any remaining foreign information. After a few hours, your crystal wands will be 'fresh and new' again. If you like, you may afterwards charge the wands up again on Rock Crystal. This activates the crystals and fortifies their effect, but is not absolutely necessary.*

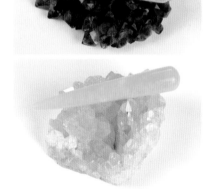

* Detailed information on the cleansing and charging of healing crystals can be found in Michael Gienger's *Purifying Crystals*, Earthdancer a Findhorn Press Imprint, 2008

Storing

Use a safe place for carefully storing your crystals. A glass-fronted cabinet is, of course, the ideal situation, but you can also carefully wrap them in fabric or keep them in small padded boxes. Crystal wands in particular are now often presented in these little boxes. Please do not lay the wands criss-cross and willy-nilly in a dish or other container, as the mutiple contacts between them will lead to a mixing of different effects. Neutral crystals, in particular, are easily "coloured" with the information from other types of crystals. This would mean that you would have to cleanse the crystals before every application. This is not necessary if you thoroughly cleanse them after each treatment and then store them carefully.

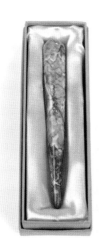

At the beginning of a treatment with crystal wands, there are two questions that need to be answered. First, what is the quickest way to find the point or the zone that will have the longest lasting effect on the presenting issue? And second, which crystal wand is suitable for this treatment? If we can answer these two questions accurately, we will get the best results possible. Certain tests have proven to be most effective for this as they directly utilise the knowledge and wisdom of the body. Muscle

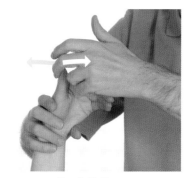

Muscle Testing

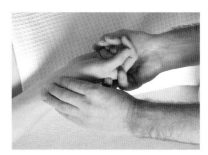

Pulse Test

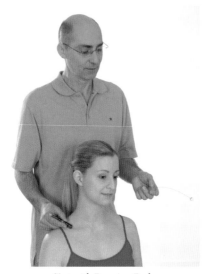

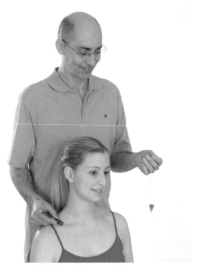

Test with Dowsing Rod *Test with a Pendulum*

testing, dowsing with a rod, dowsing with a pendulum, and the pulse test are the simplest and most effective procedures.

These methods of testing have long traditions and well-documented backgrounds with a wealth of literature to refer to, so I have avoided going into great detail here. I will restrict myself to a brief presentation of three user-friendly 'yes–no' tests, with which you can achieve good results. For further research, I recommend the literature available in your bookstore.

With all the procedures, before beginning the test we have to determine the indicators for 'yes' and 'no'. This procedure is called 'calibration', and it entails asking the client about positive and negative experiences and then observing the body's responses. These tests utilize contact with the subconscious. It is therefore extremely important that we mentally clear ourselves before the test and do not expect any particular result. Otherwise we will obtain the answers we want and not those deeply required by the person being treated. In addition, we must always ask first, before each test, whether we are actually allowed to ask this type of question. And after every test result, we owe the subconscious mind of the person being treated a 'thank you' for its willingness to communicate. It should never be taken for granted when a person opens up the depths of their psyche to such probing; through respect and gratitude for this process we obtain a better connection with clearer answers.

With all treatments and tests, we obtain the best results if we breathe along with the person we are treating. Therefore, during your treatments, always halt briefly, pay attention to the breathing rhythm of the person you are treating and tune your own breathing to theirs.

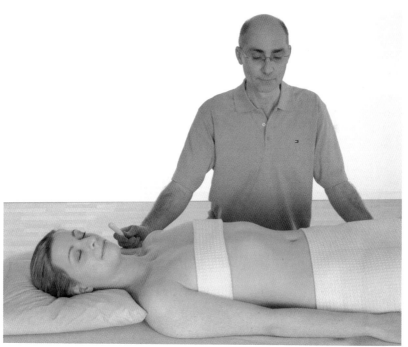

Tuning Into the Breathing Rhythm

The Muscle Test

Since kinesiology is a wide field of knowledge, this muscle test should never be used in any way other than a simple, but very useful, 'yes'–'no' test. In principle, every muscle is suitable for this test, as the agreement/rejection response always encompasses the whole person. However, we have found that we obtain the clearest signals using the thumb or the big toe.

After calibrating, ask for the information you will need in order to proceed with the test; for example, 'Which of these crystal wands is most suitable for this treatment?' or 'Is the pointed

---

Muscle Test: Calibrating

So that the person you are treating will know what you are looking for, push with a little bit of pressure against their thumb nail or big toe nail, while asking them to lightly resist the pressure. Then let go again. This is not some kind of measure of strength, so only apply a very little pressure. More is not necessary.

After your internal breath tuning, begin by asking your client for a clear, agreeing 'yes'. To do this, ask her to imagine she is sitting at a table and that her favourite dish is placed, piping hot, in front of her. Allow a few moments for the image to emerge, and when you see that the look on her face indicates that she is enjoying the dish, or if you perceive a nod, then say, 'Please test now' and press lightly for 1-3 seconds (no longer!) against the thumb or the big toe. You will then notice that the thumb or big toe of the patient remains stable in its joint and holds steady against the pressure. Then thank her and let go again. In this manner, you have obtained the 'yes' signal via a strong muscle response.

Then ask your patient for a clear, rejecting 'no'. To do this, ask her to imagine something she really does not like at all, that she finds distasteful, or even ask her to imagine a situation in which she felt weak. Please do not ask about people or events as doing so may evoke annoyance or other strong emotions, which will in turn cause defensive mechanisms to mobilize and, paradoxically, elicit a 'yes' signal. Look for the body's expression and then say 'please test now' and press briefly (1-3 seconds) against the thumb or the big toe. You will notice that the

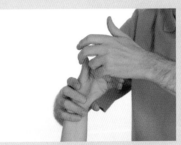

Test Indication 'Yes' –
The Thumb Holds Firm!

end or the rounded end of the crystal best for this point?' or 'In which direction should I massage to obtain the best possible balance? In this way, you will obtain clear answers from your client for their own treatment.

thumb or the big toe of the patient bends at the joint. Thus you have obtained a 'no' via a weak muscle response.

You now have clear 'yes' and 'no' signals. Next, after asking permission to continue, ask, 'Is it acceptable for us to test in this fashion?' Again saying 'please test now', apply light pressure on the thumb or the big toe. If a 'no' comes up, we have to respect it and choose a different way of proceeding.

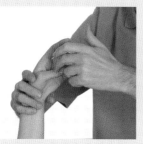

Test Indication 'No' –
The Thumb Gives Way!

After the relevant signals have been clearly established and we have permission to conduct the test, we can begin with the actual testing. The example we wish to present here is a testing procedure for selecting a crystal wand for treatment.

The first step is to determine the overall energy direction for the treatment. The question to be asked is whether energy should be conducted in, conducted away, or whether this should be an energetically neutral treatment. So, start by holding the client's thumb or big toe and asking, 'What treatment do you need?' Then go through each of the three possibilities, and after each one remember to say, 'Please test now'. 'Conducting energy in?' (Please test now). 'Conducting energy away?' (Please test now). 'Neutral?' (Please test now). If the contact is good, the answers will be very clear; when the direction of energy is correct the joint will remain firm; with the other options it will bend. If the answer is not so clear, simply attune yourself to the patient's breathing once again and repeat the three tests.

Let us assume, for argument's sake, that the patient requires more energy in this treatment. Simply select about 3–5 crystal wands that would conduct energy in (no more!), and place them one after the other on the body. The best place is above the breastbone, but if you happen to be sitting at the patient's feet, then allow yourself to be drawn to a place that feels right. ➤➤

Asking the question, 'Which of these 3 (or 4 or 5) wands would best suit this treatment?', touch the chosen place with each one of them with the request, 'Please test now'. The joint will bend with each of the unsuitable wands, but will remain firm for the suitable one; naturally this should be followed by a brief 'thank you'.

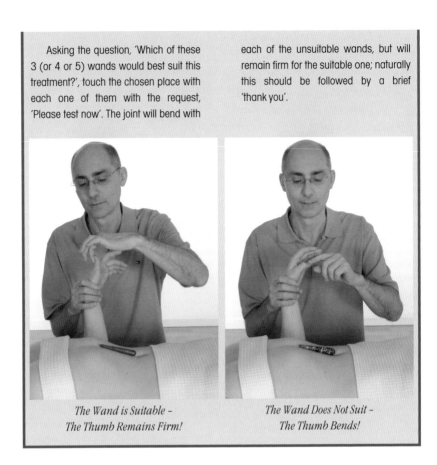

The Wand is Suitable -
The Thumb Remains Firm!

The Wand Does Not Suit -
The Thumb Bends!

Pendulum and Dowsing Rods

Dowsing rods and the pendulum are often dismissively associated with 'magic', unjustly so. It is true to say that there are certain possibilities bound up with these tools that go far beyond our imagination. However, for what we are doing here, pendulums and dowsing rods are highly reliable and simple aids for performing clear 'yes' and 'no' tests.

And an added benefit, they can be used alongside what we call 'minimal clues'. The latter are subconscious changes in posture, facial expression, breathing frequency, or movements, with which we express our own internal psychic states. If we are excited and joyful, the eye area opens up, dimples appear at the corners of the mouth, and the complexion has a slight rosy tinge. The body becomes firmer, we lift our shoulders and our breathing becomes deeper. If we receive a sad message, the 'minimal clues' look quite different: the skin becomes paler, the lips lose their fullness and the corners of the mouth sink sideways and downward. The entire body's posture loses its firmness.

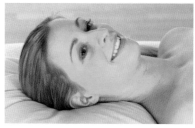

'Minimal Clues' Relating to Joy and Happiness

These reactions also apply to the 'yes–no' answers with which the client answers our questions. Usually we perceive these 'minimal clues' subconsciously as they are by nature subtle. Using a dowsing rod or a pendulum, these signals are transmitted by the micro-movements of our hands and amplified by the pendulum or rod. Thus these tools of perception resonate, and we can more easily observe the unconscious information that might otherwise be lost. The dowsing rod and the pendulum are, in this sense, wonderful

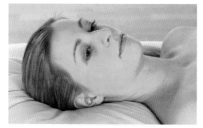

'Minimal Clues' Relating to Sadness

aids for communication with other people, those who entrust themselves to us. They also school our attentiveness.

Dowsing Rods or Pendulum Tests: Calibrating

There is a big difference between calibration for muscle testing and calibration for testing with a dowsing rod or pendulum: calibration for muscle testing consists of calibrating the reactions of the patient, whereas with a dowsing rod or pendulum we carry out the calibration on ourselves. This is because the processing of the 'yes'—'no' signals happens through our own perception when using a dowsing rod or pendulum. During this process we are in deep contact with our own subconscious, and it is therefore extremely important that we mentally clear ourselves before carrying out testing. Most failed tests with the dowsing rod or with a pendulum can be traced back to being mentally somewhere other than with the client.

So once we have paused to be sure we are fully in the here and now with our client we must begin by self-calibrating, which is done by asking about our own 'yes'–'no' reactions. Even if the dowsing rod has carried out an 'up-and-down' movement for 'yes' the last 100 times you used it, on the 101st time it may change! It is also an important step for the testing ritual. Without this self-calibrating, the test is simply a half-hearted attempt. What does 'yes' mean for me now? What does 'no' mean for me now? And what movement has the dowsing rod made in each case? Does the rod prescribe a circular motion for 'yes' or does it move up and down? Does it swing horizontally left and right for 'no', or does it begin to tremble? The more clearly we calibrate these indicators, the easier it will be for our subconscious to translate the 'minimal clues' of our client into the movements of the rod.

After calibrating, we should always ask for permission to test: 'Is it ok if we test in this manner?' Here, too, we may get a 'no', which we need to respect and go on to seek another method. If we have been given permission to continue, we can say thank you and begin the actual testing.

Dowsing Rod or Pendulum: Testing

Once permission for testing has been granted, both the testing and the questions are the same as for the muscle test.

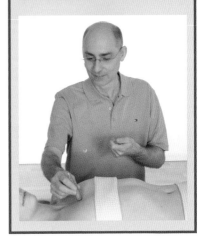

Pulse Testing

This test was developed by the French doctor Paul Nogier, and has been known under the name RAC (Reflex Auriculo Cardial) in professional circles for the last 50 years; it is considered to be a highly reliable method for asking questions of our energy systems. Pulse testing is relatively simple, but it requires a bit more sensitivity than the other two tests. With practice, this sensitivity for feeling the pulse grows astonishingly quickly. In order to be able to read the pulse quality properly and clearly, it is important that we balance

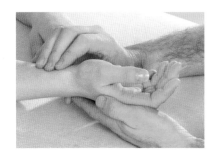

ourselves internally before testing. Otherwise we may transfer our own churned up emotions onto our client and receive the wrong results. We can balance ourselves by taking a few deep, conscious breaths, and/or performing the 'grounding' exercise on page 65.

Pulse Test: Calibrating and Testing

We usually check the pulse at the wrist. If the pulse is too weak to feel it there, the stronger pulse of the carotid artery is always available. However, be very careful not to exert any pressure. Or, with a bit of practise, we can feel the pulse in other places; for example, on the top of the foot or in the groin. Use fingers rather than the thumb to feel the pulse, otherwise it might be our own pulse we feel.

To begin with, feel for the present pulse rate without intent. Then ask for a positive reference, a 'yes', and pay attention to the change in the pulse. Note whether the pulse is faster, slower, harder, softer, or if the change is insignificant. This is the pulse signal of the patient for 'yes'. After that, we can calibrate for 'no', with a question about an unpleasantly weakening reference.

Then we can begin with the testing in the same manner as we did with the other testing procedures.

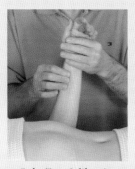

Pulse Test: Calibrating

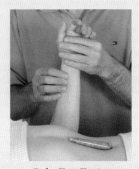

Pulse Test: Testing

Crystal Oils and Crystal Balms

The use of crystals in healing was described as far back as 2000 years ago by the Greek physician, Dioskurides, and also 800 years ago by Hildegard von Bingen. Ever since, the healing powers of the 'fruits of the Earth' have enjoyed a renaissance, and we are becoming more and more aware of their many applications. Energizing water with crystals has gained widespread acceptance because its qualities can be perceived and tasted. Oil as a carrier medium is also now gaining recognition; the avant-garde practitioners of these preparations, Monika Grund-

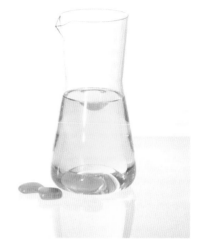

mann and Franca Bauer, have been using crystal oils for many years with great success in cosmetics and healing applications.

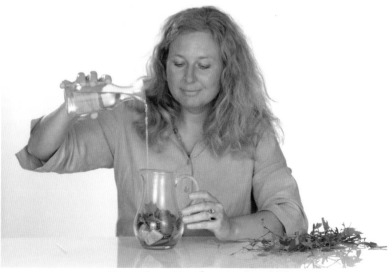

Franca Bauer Manufacturing Crystal Oils

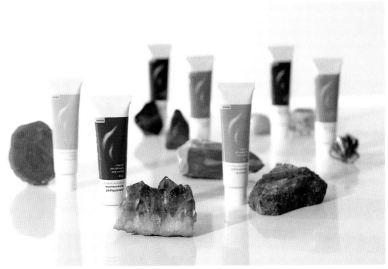

PEKANA Crystal Balms with the Crystals Used for their Preparation

A company called PEKANA took a different path. Known worldwide for its homeopathic/spagyric* healing aids, Dr. Beyersdorff and his wife have used their alchemical methods on crystals too and developed balms from them, each one carrying clear chakra and planetary references. Although they have only been available since the beginning of 2007, these crystal balms have already been tried and tested successfully. Important to note, Balm No. 2 (orange) has the wonderful 'side-effect' of firming up wrinkles in the corners of the eyes!

* Spagyrics was formulated by Paracelsus and describes a procedure for the manufacture of healing agents following basic alchemical principles.

In both crystal oils and crystal balms, the essential oils actually prepare the body and forge a pathway for absorbing crystal energies. In this manner, the energies of the crystals take effect within us in the most beneficial way, or, as Dr. Beyersdorff describes it, they create a path to holistic health.

In order to eliminate doubts about the energetic potency of crystal oils, I would like to tell you a story of the development phase of Monika Grundmann's crystal oils:

The Swiss manufacturer, Farfalla Essentials, were already running a series of tests on crystal oils and receiving positive results, when, just to be sure, the company decided to check energetic quality with a final test before beginning production. For this purpose, Farfalla sent several specimens to Monika Grundmann with a request to test the oil specimens, through dowsing (radiesthesia*), for the crystal information belonging to each oil. During the development phase, Monika Grundmann had always had the oils tested by an independent dowser. Well, there was a great commotion when her tester reported, even after multiple tests, that not a single one of the specimens contained crystal information. Monika Grundmann, now utterly irritated, passed on this report to the production manager at Farfalla. Highly gratified, the latter began with the production of the oils! It had been the expected result. After all the many tests that had gone before, the company had purposely sent Monika oil specimens without any crystal information. This way they could be entirely sure that it was possible to check whether the oils had been informed, and that the process did not rely merely on wishful thinking.

Due to their consistency, crystal oils are used mainly as energetic massage oils, while crystal balms unfold their strengths mainly in small areas of application, as in chakra treatment and point massage.

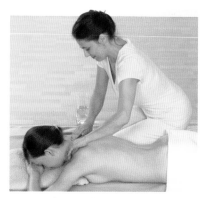

Monika Grundmann Carrying Out a Massage with Crystal Oils

The qualities of crystal oils and crystal balms make them ideal to complement crystal wand massage. For the basic massage, test for a suitable crystal oil, and then apply a crystal balm during the course of the treatment for alleviating any kind of specific interference on a certain point. Let us allow the products to speak for themselves:

* 'Radiesthesia' refers to the ability to sense or perceive waves emanating from the earth, water, other substances, or even other types of energies. The term covers all abilities generally classed as 'dowsing'.

Monika Grundmann's
Crystal Oils

The seven crystal oils developed by Monika Grundmann are manufactured using organic Jojoba oil as a base, and then three crystals are used for making each oil. Each crystal oil is then refined with suitable essential oils. The name given to the oil also indicates its area of use.

Crystal Oil 'Anti-Stress'
Crystals: Aventurine, Magnesite, Smoky Quartz
Essential Oils: Sweet Orange, Rosewood, Lavender, Ylang Ylang

Crystal Oil 'Security'
Crystals: White Agate, Nephrite, Serpentine
Essential Oils: Vanilla, Sandalwood, Benzoin Siam

Crystal Oil 'Serenity'
Crystals: Blue Quartz, Dumortierite, Magnesite
Essential Oils: Lavender, Rosewood, Mandarin, Camomile

Crystal Oil 'In the Flow'
Crystals: Sodalite, Blue Chalcedony, Amber
Essential Oils: White Fir, Geranium, Palmarosa

Crystal Oil 'Fountain of Youth'
Crystals: Green Fluorite, Chrysoprase, Peridot
Essential Oils: Juniper Berry, Sweet Fennel, Lemon

Crystal Oil 'Regeneration'
Crystals: Epidote, Ocean Agate, Zoisite with Ruby
Essential Oils: Ravensara, Myrtle, Litsea Cubeba

Particular synergy can be achieved in massage if we use a wand of the same crystal used for producing the crystal oil. But this is only a suggestion, not a restriction! Assuming they suit the issue being treated, crystal oils can, in principle, be combined with any crystal wand. Monika Grundmann's crystal oils are available from Farfalla Essentials, and in the specialist trade.

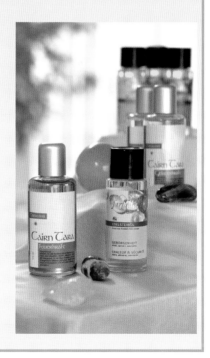

Crystal Balms by PEKANA

There are seven PEKANA crystal balms. For each balm, two crystals are pulverized down to grain sizes of 40 μm and worked into a balm base in an alchemical process with two related essential oils. The balms have the following correspondences:

PEKANA Crystal Balm 1 (dark red):
'Life Energy'
Planet: Sun
Chakra: Root Chakra
Themes: Steadfastness and Uprightness
Body: Spine, Sexual organs
Crystals: Garnet, Sugilite
Essential Oils: Rose, Spike lavender
Synergy with Crystal Wands: Basalt, Epidote, Gabbro, Hematite, Obsidian, Tiger Iron, Zoisite

PEKANA Crystal Balm 2 (orange):
'Openness'
Planet: Moon
Chakra: Sacral Chakra
Themes: Dissolving sadness and acquiring patience
Body: Abdomen, Back, Joints
Crystals: Jasper, Emerald
Essential Oils: Rosemary, Cedar Wood
Synergy with Crystal Wands: Apatite, Aragonite, Dolomite, Jasper, Marble, Mookaite, Onyx

PEKANA Crystal Balm 3 (yellow):
'Harmony'
Planet: Mars
Chakra: Solar Plexus

Themes: Alleviating psychological wounds and restoring harmony
Body: Stomach, Liver, Gall bladder, Spleen, Pancreas
Crystals: Carnelian, Onyx
Essential Oils: Bergamot, Cypress
Synergy with Crystal Wands: Bronzite, orange Calcite, Carnelian, Ocean Agate, Tiger's Eye, Fossil Wood

PEKANA Crystal Balm 4 (green): 'Joy'
Planet: Mercury
Chakra: Heart Chakra
Themes: Attaining a peaceful heart and inner wisdom
Body: Heart
Crystals: Jade, Tourmaline
Essential Oils: Sandalwood, Rosewood
Synergy with Crystal Wands: Amazonite, Heliotrope, Nephrite, Rhodonite, Rose Quartz, Serpentine

PEKANA Crystal Balm 5 (mid-blue): 'Trust'
Planet: Jupiter
Chakra: Throat Chakra
Themes: Easing communication, and creating clarity
Body: Front of neck and head area
Crystals: Chalcedony, Rock Crystal
Essential Oils: Peppermint, Sage
Synergy with Crystal Wands: Aquamarine, Rock Crystal, Chalcedony, Dumortierite, Moss Agate, Snow Quartz

PEKANA Crystal Balm 6 (dark blue):
'Clarity'
Planet: Venus
Chakra: Brow Chakra (third eye)

Themes: Dissolving blockages, and acquiring peace
Body: Centre of forehead, kidney area
Crystals: Sodalite, Agate
Essential Oils: Camomile (blue), Orange peel
Synergy with Crystal Wands: Agate, Blue Quartz, white Feldspar, Labradorite, Lapis Lazuli, Sodalite

PEKANA Crystal Balm 7 (violet):
'Cleansing'
Planet: Saturn
Chakra: Crown Chakra
Themes: Opening the chakra above the head and creating protection

Body: Neck, sides of the neck and throat, skin
Crystals: Amethyst, green Aventurine
Essential Oils: Lavender, Cypress
Synergy with Crystal Wands: Amethyst, green Aventurine, Eldarite, Fluorite, Lepidolite, Tourmaline (Schorl)

The 'Synergy with Crystal Wands' aspect listed for each balm is intended as a suggestion only, not as a restriction! PEKANA crystal balms are available in the specialist trade and from selected pharmacies.

When using combinations of crystal wands with crystal oils or crystal balms, there are three different kinds of applications: 'similar', 'additional' and 'complementary'.

In a 'similar' application, we use oils and balms with wands that represent similar themes or have similar effects. This creates a mutual amplification of the desired effects.

In an 'additional' application, we extend the effect of the massage by combining crystal wands with oils and balms that have a different effect. A successful combination of this kind extends the range of possibilities.

In a 'complementary' application we combine crystal wands with oils and balms that have the opposite effect. In this way, with a little bit of sensitivity, we are able to carry out a deeply effective and balancing massage. The contrary aspects will initially bring a little more tension to the application, but will then create a balance that leaves all possibilities open. The rest is up to us; for example, the manner in which we carry out the massage, or how we massage.

Combining crystal wands with crystal oils and crystal balms enriches enormously the range of possibilities and results when giving a massage treatment. It is really worth becoming familiar with them.

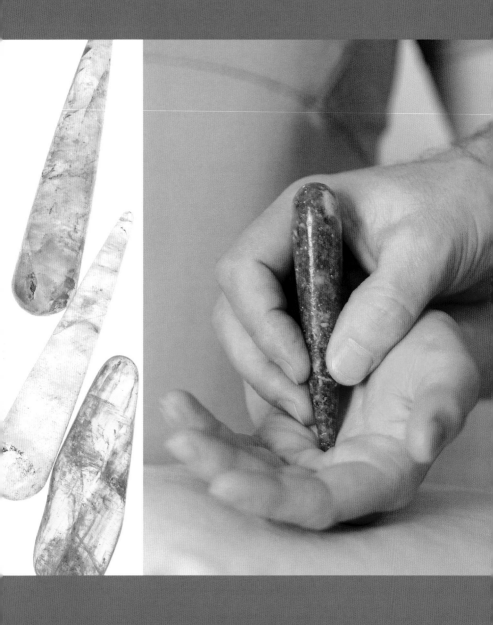

Massage with Crystal Wands

Touching is a basic human need. At some point, millions of years ago, our ancestors must have discovered that mutual grooming did not simply remove lice, fleas and other parasites, but that touch also alleviated pain. It is no wonder then that we have, over the course of time, perfected an unbeliev-

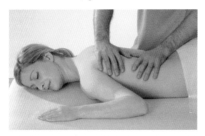

Classic Massage

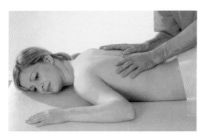

Shiatsu Massage

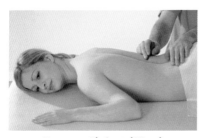

Massage with Crystal Wands

able variety of hands-on applications. Massage, chiropractic, physiotherapy, Shaitsu, the energetic laying on of hands – all manual treatments have their roots in mutual touching, and are actually all forms of massage, in which we use our hands as healing tools.

With the decoding of our genes it became clear that not only our eye colour or body structure are genetically based, but that fundamental abilities are also inherited. Thus we do not need to learn how to grasp a stone or a branch. The development of a child from crawling to an upright walking posture also follows genetic rules. Like-wise the need to touch each other belongs to our most ancient human make up. Seen in this way, the ability to massage has also been with us from the cradle, and it is up to us whether we encourage this ability or allow it to fade.

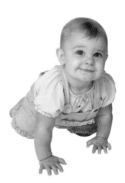

Crawling Comes 'All By Itself!

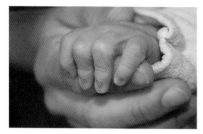

Touching - An Ancient Need...

Another piece of evolutionary equipment that lies dormant within us, and is awaiting its wake-up call, is sensitivity to energies. Cats prefer to lie over water veins; ants erect their anthills preferably over crossing points of earth currents; the fact that dogs would never sleep on such high-energy locations – abilities like these are present everywhere in the animal kingdom. We too sense when the energy feels right in a place, and when it does not. It is not only Australian Aborigines and South African Bushmen who have this kind of sensitivity. Our water diviners and dowsers also provide evidence that these talents are still present in the modern world.

An example of this was my father, who, while visiting his two sons in South Africa, found precisely the spot where water could be sourced. The story began when our neighbours at the Cape of Good Hope wanted to dig for a well, and our father offered to find a suitable location for them. Geologists had previously located two general areas, each measuring about ten metres in diameter, where there

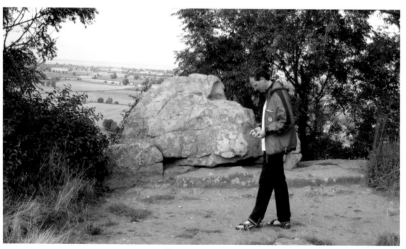

Dowser in Action

63

was the greatest likelihood of finding water, at an unspecified depth. Now, we know that when one is digging a well it is crucial to hit the right point. One metre out of place and there will be no water. Without any kind of previous information, our father set out with his dowsing rod to search, and he found places in each of the two areas. With the first one, which he favoured, he said that the water was at a depth of 34 metres; however, one would have to dig through a seven-metre-thick layer of rock at a depth of 22 metres. He also thought that the capacity of the borehole would be about 1,000 litres per hour. When our neighbours began boring at the designated spot, the workers wanted to stop boring when they reached the rock layer, at the depth my father had indicated. Naturally, our neighbours pushed to carry on. When he got back to Germany, my father was informed that he had erred by one metre depth and by 100 litres of water capacity. News of this success story spread, and soon my father received a number of further invitations to look for wells. Unfortunately, his state of health did not allow him to continue.

Deep down we all have a 'feel' for what is good for us and what will harm us.

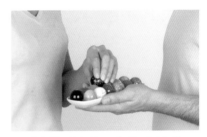

Intuitive Selection of a Crystal Ball

And all of us have our own 'energy world' at our disposal. Some of us sense energies from the Earth, some have access to human energy fields, some are able to sense the energies in a room. It is a curious fact, however, that all humans are able to sense the energies of crystals. Often this is restricted to intuitively reaching for a certain crystal rather than another. This can be clearly demonstrated with the Joya® balls, which are all the same size and all tempered the same way. If you allow someone to root around with closed eyes in a group of balls, even sceptics will select, again and again, those with similar qualities. No wonder then that massages with crystal wands 'speak to' deep levels of our humanness. The compass for this type of massage is simply our own intuition – our sensed knowledge.

Naturally it is therefore even more important that we as practitioners tune in to these inner qualities and open up our portals of awareness to them. The following exercise, which has been tried and tested countless times, can be carried out in moments or can be expanded into a wonderful meditation.

Remember, crystals bring the gift of joie de vivre. Please do this little exercise with an inward smile!

Sit down comfortably, with your feet firmly on the ground, and lay your hands on your navel.

Now imagine that your feet are taking root. With every breath, feel the rising and falling of your tummy under your hands, and feel the roots spreading out further and deeper into the Earth. Keep sending your roots down, down and down, until they reach the core of the Earth, right to the magma. Allow your roots to enjoy splashing around in the magma, and watch as all burdening thoughts and feelings flow away.

Now please bring your attention to the top of your head. Imagine you are opening your spiritual 'sunroof', and then search in the starry sky for a beautiful star. Allow that star to shine down on you, and feel how this very pleasurable light is streaming down your spine and flowing down through your root tips into the magma. Gradually, this light will begin spraying like a sparkling bubble bath of light around your roots.

In this way, you are creating a beautiful, light-flooded connection between our outer universe and your inner Earth, and you will feel how good it is to be a mediator of energies. This will solidly anchor you to your place in the present. Feel how all the burdening energies are flowing away and are being transformed through this connection. If you can make space to experience this 'flow', you will be able to begin giving your treatment in a fresh and composed state of mind.

Beginning the Massage

At the beginning of a massage the aim is to get to know your client holistically, to get to know the person who has entrusted himself or herself to you, and to give them the opportunity to see you as a companion in their experience. The treatment then begins by making contact with the person's body, perhaps by quietly taking his or her feet in your hands for a few moments, or holding their shoulders, or laying a hand on their tummy. This mutual perceiving of each other is also a welcome opportunity to breathe deeply and tune in to your client's breathing pattern. Even if it lasts only a few moments, these are often the decisive moments for the whole treatment. The person being treated will feel 'accepted' in the fullest sense of the word.

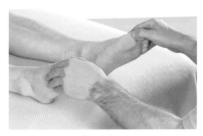

Making Contact

After the 'tuning in', follow your own intuition and choose a crystal wand to begin stroking down from the neck to the pelvis. If you are massaging within the reflex zones, the first stroking should be through the zones from the neck down to the pelvic area. This stroking action can be combined with the use of a massage oil. According to the mood, you may want to choose a crystal oil from those described in the previous chapter.

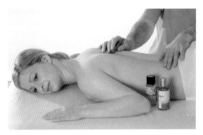

Crystal Wand with Crystal Oil

Position of the Hands

Hold the crystal wand in a relaxed manner as if it were a writing implement, or place a fingertip on the end of the crystal that leads the point of contact with your client's body. The shape of the wand will allow you to guide it and exert the right amount of pressure, even with oily fingers. Think of the wand as an extended finger through which you can feel 'into' the client's skin. If you allow your breath to flow right down to the end of the crystal wand, with a little practical experience you will be able to feel the tissue with all its qualities, just as if you were touching the skin with your bare hands.

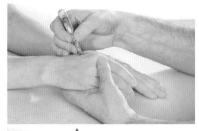

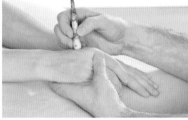

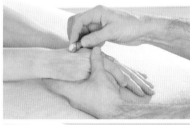

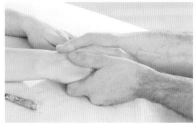

Follow your intuition and inner perception. Sometimes you will apply the rounded end of the crystal wand, some-times the pointed end; sometimes you will massage flatly with the side of the crystal, and sometimes you will work with your hands alone. Allow yourself to be guided by your hands on an inner level, while paying particular attention to the following:

◎ Always remain in physical contact with your client. One hand should always maintain that contact so that your client feels comfortable and safe.

◎ A massage with or without crystal wands should *never* feel unpleas-ant, let alone painful. The measur-ing stick for the wellbeing of the client should be the depth of their breath. If your client breathes deeply, you are on the right track. If their breathing becomes shallow, you should change the intensity of your hold; usually this means becoming more sensitive to the other person.

◎ All applications with crystal wands require slow treatment techniques, which will suit the rhythm of your client's breathing.

◎ Always work from your own centre. To help with this, imagine you are a Sumo-wrestler weighing 200kg. You would then be standing or kneeling next to your client and breathing into the centre of your body just beneath your navel. The Japanese believe this is the point where lies the *hara*. If you allow your massage holds to emerge out of the hara, you will experience a much greater intensity while expending a minimum amount of energy. In this way your treatments will become more pleasant, more adapted to the mood, and clearly more effective.

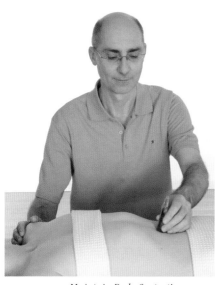

Maintain Body Contact!

Toning and Sedating

One subject that always plays a large part in massage with crystal wands is the amount of energy being conducted in and the amount of energy being conducted away from any given point on the body. Conducting energy IN is called 'toning'. Conducting energy AWAY is called 'sedating'. Deciding which is needed is made easy by the shape of the wand and its subsequent testability. The tip of the wand bundles energies and the round end conducts them away. Thus, if we place the tip on a certain point and it tests strongly as 'yes', then we know that additional energy is required there. If we get a positive signal at the rounded end, we can be certain that this point requires energy to be conducted away. (The 'yes'-'no' testing method is described in the previous chapter.)

We can also look to the qualities of the crystals themselves when making decisions about a treatment. A number of crystals, such as red Jasper, Basalt, or orange Calcite, are veritable power bombs, while others, such as Aventurine, Amethyst or Sodalite, have an immediately noticeable calming and balancing effect.

Making choices regarding a suitable crystal wand usually happens at the beginning of a treatment, and applies

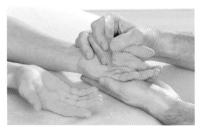

Toning

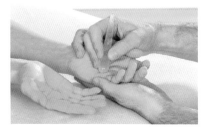

Sedating

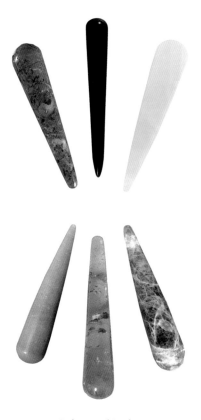

Stokers and Strokers

for the entire treatment, whereas whether we use the tip or the rounded end can vary from point to point. In individual cases, a point on the body may even require a special crystal quality. If in doubt, test for the answer.

During the course of a treatment, you may soon discover that probing and stroking massage movements will merge seamlessly with each other and alternate as needed. In essence, three movements will be used in the massage: stroking, circling, and 'basic unblocking'.

Strokes

For all stroking movements, a few drops of massage oil are required so that your hands glide easily across the skin. Please use only a few drops though, otherwise you may lose a sense of contact with the client. Stroking is meant to be slow, thereby allowing you to follow along with the breathing of the client and to stop if their breathing changes or even halts. Usually the rounded end of the crystal wand is used for stroking movements. This does not, however, apply to stroking conducted along the acupressure meridians, which is usually done using the pointed tip of the crystal.

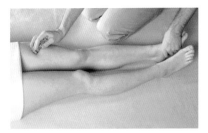

Stroking the Muscles

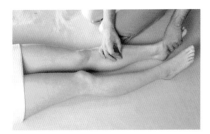

Stroking along the Meridians

The most frequent 'longways' stroking is carried out along the back, either side of the spine. Stroking upwards has an activating effect; stroking downwards has a balancing effect. Please avoid stroking along the central line on top of the spinal projections. With the exception of a very few therapeutic applications, you should also not cross over the central line of the spine.

On the front of the body other principles are applicable when using crystal wands: only stroke upward, from the pelvis up to the neck. Never stroke from the top downwards on the front of the body as this will lead to an undesirable opening of the energy field of the client, which is usually perceived by them as unpleasant. Naturally, this may be welcomed within the framework of a loving massage.

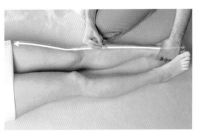

Balancing Stroking

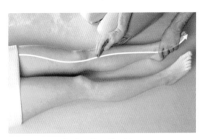

Activating Stroking

In addition to 'longways' stroking, there are three special types of stroking: circular stroking, spiral circling and sunray stroking.

Circular Stroking

This technique is often applied to the face, where we use the rounded ends of two (of the same type!) crystal wands to make parallel circling movements around the face. This is wonderful for dissolving facial tension. Monika Grundmann has described these applications in detail in her book, *Crystal Balance.** Naturally, circular movements are also very pleasant on whichever part of the body is being massaged.

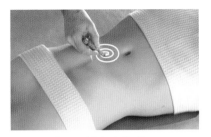

Inward Spiral Circling

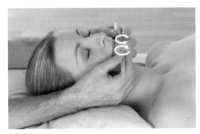

Circular Stroking

Spiral Circling

Inward turning spiral movements concentrate energy from an area with a diameter of about 5-7cm into a single point; this is generally achieved using the tip of a wand. Such 'bundling' enables us to rebuild energy deficits.

Sunray Stroking

This application is always required if we come across points or zones that demonstrate an excess of energy. As if you were tracing the rays of a sun, stroke outwards with the round end of the crystal wand; this distributes excess energy into the surrounding area.

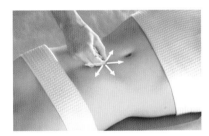

Sunrays

Before using the spiral circling and sunray techniques, you should always carry out a basic unblocking of the point (see page 73). That is the only way to guarantee a lasting effect.

* Monika Grundmann, *Crystal Balance*, Earthdancer a Findhorn Press Imprint, 2008

Circling on the Spot

This massage technique can be both investigative and therapeutic, and, depending on the intensity, will have a stimulating, neutral or calming effect. For this procedure, use the rounded end of the crystal wand to circle around one point, always remaining in contact with the skin, without sliding. After about 5-7 circles, move to the next point, overlapping with the previous massage circle as you go.

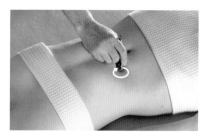

Circling on the Spot

Quick holds with more intense pressure applied are activating. Slow, gentle holds are balancing.

This hold can be used to feel out the structures of the connective tissue under the skin. It can also be used as a massage hold to spread relaxation into the surrounding tissue after the basic unblocking procedure, or to tone the tissue. Please carry out these circling movements very slowly, in time with the breathing rhythm of your client.

If we follow our intuition, the direction of movement of these circles is generally unimportant. However, if you should sense an inner resistance to a direction, or sense tension, or you notice an autonomic reaction in your client, simply change directions.

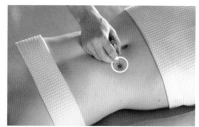

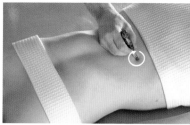

Change Direction if Resistance is Detected!

One very pleasant application is to use two of the same kind of crystal wand to move in parallel from the top to the bottom of the spine, with one on the left side of the spine, one on the right. The first stroke should be about two fingers' width away from the central line, the next stroke should be two fingers' width further away, and so on.

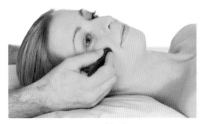

Basic Unblocking

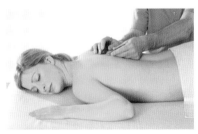

Balancing Autonomic Reactions

Basic Unblocking Procedure

When treating with crystal wands, one of the most important procedures of all is 'basic unblocking'. In order for an energy disruption in a point or zone to become capable of reacting, it is neces-sary to respect that which is being treated. Using a technique called 'basic unblocking', we can respectfully obtain affirmation from the client of acceptance for change.

'Basic unblocking' is a very simple technique. Just remain quietly on one point with the rounded end of a crystal wand, using emphatic and consistent pressure (below the pain threshold!), until the tension, and thus the unpleasant sensation, decreases. You will experience the wand sinking into the skin and the client clearly breathing deeply, often combined with a sigh. This is a signal that you are in contact with the client's body awareness, and that you have permission from those deeper levels of being to proceed further. Basic unblocking is, so to speak, a conversation with the client's inner healing wisdom and 'health guardians'.

Imagine that you are going on holiday for a few days and you have left your house key with a good friend so

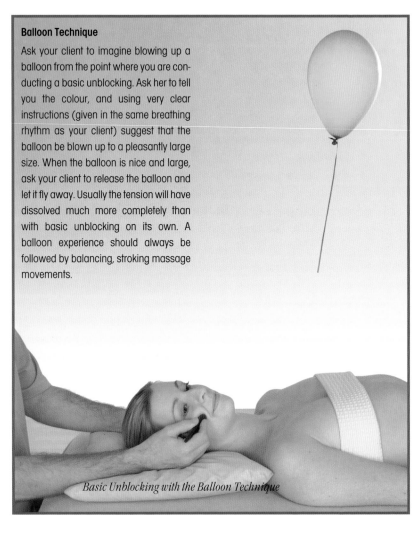

Balloon Technique

Ask your client to imagine blowing up a balloon from the point where you are conducting a basic unblocking. Ask her to tell you the colour, and using very clear instructions (given in the same breathing rhythm as your client) suggest that the balloon be blown up to a pleasantly large size. When the balloon is nice and large, ask your client to release the balloon and let it fly away. Usually the tension will have dissolved much more completely than with basic unblocking on its own. A balloon experience should always be followed by balancing, stroking massage movements.

Basic Unblocking with the Balloon Technique

that he can water your plants. As he wishes to be particularly kind to you, and you have recently talked of renovating your kitchen, he uses this opportunity to wallpaper your kitchen in your absence. He does the job perfectly, with a pattern of wallpaper *he* finds amazing – blue elephants with pink dots on a vivid green background. When you arrive back home he greets you at the door with a beaming smile and immediately shows you his accomplishment.

How enthusiastic would you be about his well-intentioned gesture? It is the same if we approach a treatment with the best intention and assume that we know what the client needs. If our dear friend had only asked, we would have told him what kind of wallpaper we would prefer. Now we feel put upon and faced with a dilemma. Should we honour his good intention or should we chase him out of the house and end the friendship?

Basic unblocking helps us keep friends, and clients. In this procedure we use the client's physical reactions to question them about their wishes, and to ensure that the 'return from the holiday' is a pleasant one and that everyone concerned will be delighted with the 'new kitchen' for a long time to come.

Especially with energetic techniques such as reflexology, acupressure or chakra treatment, basic unblocking ensures greater attention to the needs of the body and the soul. This can also be deepened with breathing techniques. Often, basic unblocking with a suitable crystal wand in connection with the 'balloon technique' is sufficient to induce an overall feeling of wellbeing.

Free Intuitive Massage

From the elements described in the previous sections, you can create a 'free' intuitive massage for the entire body or for certain areas of the body.

When massaging, always follow your intuition and ability to empathize. If you have a clear intention to do something good for the client and you always remain in physical contact, you will sense what is good for him or her. Remain in the same breathing rhythm as you client and pay attention to their subtle signals (facial expression, physical tension, posture, reactions). Allow your hands to lead you, and massage generously and with appropriate pressure. Such an intuitive massage will do your client the world of good, and you too!

As an alternative to intuitive massage, after beginning the massage you may also progress to one of the special applications described in the following chapter.

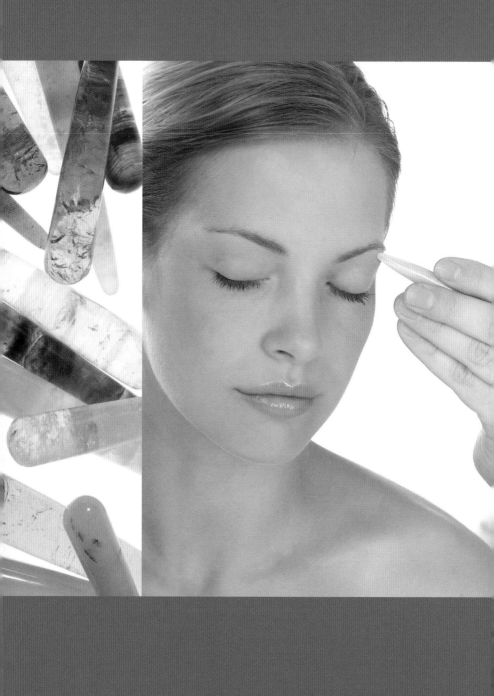

Applications

In the past twelve years, crystal wands have been increasingly employed in a wide range of applications and have been tried and tested successfully in acupressure, meridian massage, chakra treatment, and other energy massage techniques. In the following, I would like to illuminate further the possibilities of these energetic tools in five massage treatment programmes:

- for Wellness
- for Relaxation
- for Energy
- for Beauty and Love
- for Energetic Protection

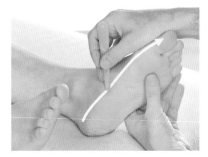

Power Massage

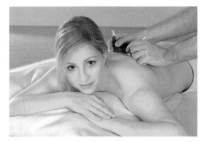

Beauty and Love Massage

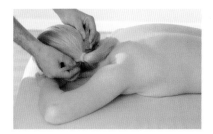

Wellness Massage

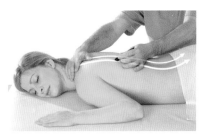

Protective Massage

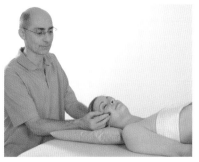

Relaxation Massage

Naturally, crystal wands open up even more possibilities. The programme titles refer to therapeutic applications, although the boundaries for wellbeing treatments are quite fluid. For further treatments we should mention in particular reflex zone massage with crystal wands. That is why I have gone into more depth with respect to the contribution from the book, *Crystal Massage for Health and Healing.* *

Usually oil is an integral part of a massage. The skin becomes smoother for the hands to glide across and holds can be carried out more 'fluidly'. For some time now, crystal oils and crystal balms have been available for use in massage (see 'Basics' chapter), and I am pleased to incorporate them into the following treatment programmes. The effects of the treatments are clearly deepened with the help of crystal oils and balms.

The Wellness Programme

Wellness goes beyond good health and a feeling of wellbeing. It is a desire for the 'pleasurable silence of the organs' (Hans-Georg Gadamer)** and means bringing the body and the soul into a pleasant and stable union. We need this especially if we are experiencing lack of enthusiasm, tiredness, or are feeling unwell.

* Michael Gienger, *Crystal Massage for Health and Healing*, Earthdancer a Findhorn Press Imprint, 2006
** Hans-Georg Gadamer, *The Enigma of Health: The Art of Healing in a Scientific Age*, Stanford University Press, 1996

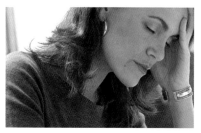

Lack of Enthusiasm, Tiredness and Feeling Unwell

For this situation, massage with crystal wands will help support the three great systems in the body – the nervous system, the metabolism and the motoric system. Crystal healing gives us clear indications for what is needed: Dumortierite stabilizes the connections of the body and the psyche, Fossil Wood stimulates the metabolism, and Bloodstone provides supportive impulses for the coordination of movements. Naturally, additional crystals are available for each one of these areas. The qualities of the additional crystals are described in detail in the crystal wand portraits in the 'Basics' chapter.

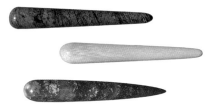

A typical 'Wellness Set': Dumortierite, Fossil Wood, Bloodstone

A central concern with all treatments relates to the harmonisation of the body and soul. We know of sufficient examples where it becomes clear that psychological events are triggering physical reactions. If we feel sadness, we feel low and depressed; we hang our heads and our shoulders droop. However, if we feel we are in love then we feel confident, our bodies have good muscle tone, and we have almost unlimited reserves of energy at our disposal. Improving the quality of these psychosomatic junction points is one of the outstanding abilities of crystals. We know of a number of these junction points at which the body and the psyche contact each other and exert a strong influence on each other.

Psychosomatic Junction Points (a selection)

Breath Reference
Breathing is connected with all life and mind functions. If we are excited or nervous we breathe faster, and breathing techniques provide a deep sense of relaxation in all types of meditation.

Immune System
The immune response can be influenced by thoughts and inner images. This realisation is successfully employed by 'psycho-neural immunology' in alternative cancer treatment.

Hormones Relating to Sexual Arousal
The neuropeptides, as they are correctly referred to, possess receptors not only in the brain, but also in many other tissues; for example, in the immune system and in the sphincter muscles.

Proprioception
The sensory receptors of our joints are responsible for our human upright posture as they control muscle tension. This, in turn, also governs our 'posture' in the psychological sense.

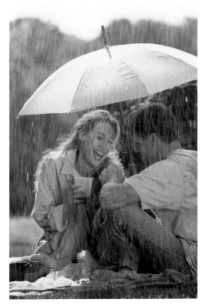

In Love

The crystal most able to support this inner communication at the psycho-somatic junction points is Dumortierite. This 'take it easy' crystal stimulates the life energies and lends composure. Apart from that, Dumotierite also clearly relaxes masseurs! We may also use other crystals as alternatives to this crystal, e.g. Rock Crystal, Obsidian, Rose Quartz, or Serpentine. Further crystal wands are described in the portraits in the 'Basics' chapter.

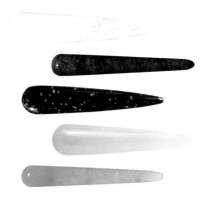

Rock Crystal, Dumortierite, Snowflake Obsidian, Rose Quartz, Serpentine

The Metabolism

Another basic requirement for the 'pleasurable silence of the organs' is a properly functioning metabolism. How often we hear the term 'metabolism', and yet how few of us are able to conjure up a picture of it. But it is really quite simple:

In order for our organism with its 50 billion cells to function optimally, all the cells have to be supplied properly with what they need. For this task, evolution has had the genius to equip us with so-called 'basic regulation'. In brief, this means that all of our cells are as though bathed in a kind of internal 'ancient ocean' from which each cell obtains all it needs for life. In the tissue fluids between the cells, the blood vessels deposit oxygen and nutrients, and it is also from there that the waste products are transported away. That which is expelled from the cells is picked up by the lymph system from the 'ancient ocean' and conducted into the internal recycling system. Basically, it is this exchange that we usually call the 'metabolism'.

In this 'basic regulation' system, reflexology and other treatments work like an egg whisk that whirls around in the deposited waste matter. The waste then needs to be expelled out of the system as quickly as possible by drinking

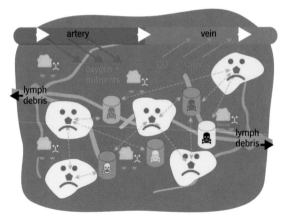

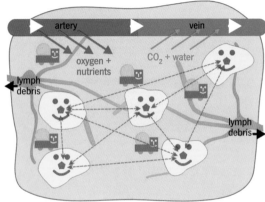

Metabolism and 'Basic Regulation'

plenty of fluids such as water or herbal teas. Otherwise the client will experience unpleasant treatment reactions such as tiredness, irritability, or an increase in existing symptoms. If we can clear the metabolic system, the cells are able to communicate better with each other and have optimal conditions in which to work. In such a 'basic regulation' system the impulse provided by crystal massage is to unfold and improve the interplay of the cells within the entire metabolic process.

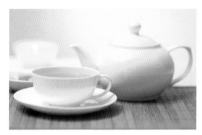

Tea or Water Support the Massage

A Basic Massage for the Improvement of Psychosomatic Tuning

Use a Dumortierite crystal wand, or another suitable crystal wand (test for the right one), along the spinal column about 3-5 times on the left and the same on the right, moving down from the back of the neck to the pelvic area. Through this the client will experience a better basic mood and be able to accept the further impulses more easily.

The treatment that follows will depend on whether the client requires stimulation or relaxation (if in doubt, test).

If the treatment is to be stimulating, move in small circular movements (about 4–5 per location), starting below in the pelvic area upwards towards the neck. Use the pointed end of the crystal wand for this, and ensure that the direction of the circular movements proceeds towards the spine. This will also apply if carrying out this tuning on the feet or the hands.

For a calming or relaxing treatment, the circular movements should be carried out with the round end of the crystal, and in the other direction. Therefore, start at the top at the neck and proceed downwards, with the circular movements directing away from the spine.

On the back, these massages are most effective if carried out with two wands of the same type of crystal in parallel. If massaging with one hand, the free hand accompanies the movements of the other side. If you are treating the feet or hands, hold the area being treated with one hand, and then massage the reflex zones (at the spinal areas in question), one after the other. It is not important which hand or foot we start with. During this treatment 'journey', carry out a basic unblocking procedure at the noticeable points and then carry on as normal.

After one of these Wellness treatments, flat moods will be lifted, nervous tension will give way to a more pleasant state, and the client will experience an extremely pleasant 'tuning' of the organs and the body.

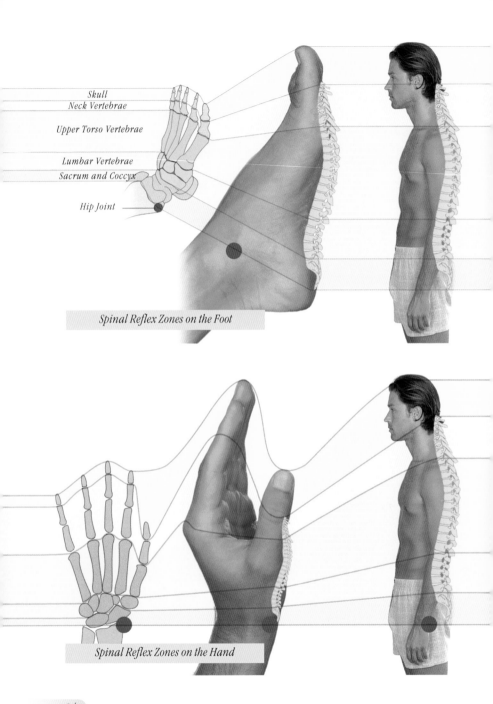

Skull
Neck Vertebrae

Upper Torso Vertebrae

Lumbar Vertebrae
Sacrum and Coccyx

Hip Joint

Spinal Reflex Zones on the Foot

Spinal Reflex Zones on the Hand

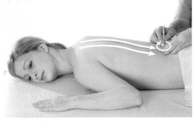

Psychosomatic Basic Massage with Two Crystal Wands

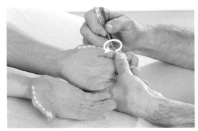

Psychosomatic Basic Massage with One Crystal Wand

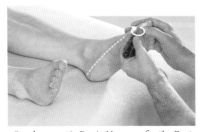

Psychosomatic Basic Massage for the Hand

Psychosomatic Basic Massage for the Foot

Stimulating the Metabolism

After tuning in (preferably with a Dumortierite wand), ask your client to turn over. While this is happening, change over to using a 'metabolic crystal'. Using this crystal, massage generously but gently, in sequence, the areas of the foot governing the intestines, the belly and the hands. As with nearly all applications, take care of problem areas with a basic unblocking and then finally stroke-massage with sunray movements.

Afterwards, proceed to the movement integration procedure, and then carry out the de-tuning stroking massage at the end.

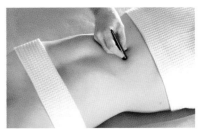

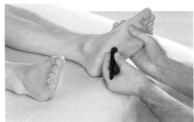

Massage of the Intestinal Reflex Zones

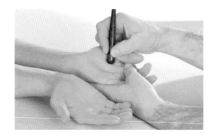

For stimulation of the metabolism, preferably use crystal wands made of Fossil Wood, Rose Quartz or Red Jasper. See also the crystal wand portraits in the 'Basics' chapter for other alternatives.

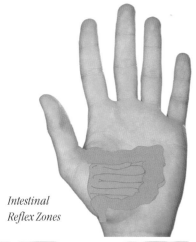

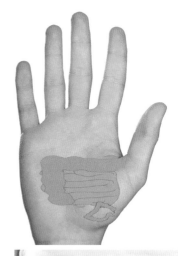

*Intestinal
Reflex Zones*

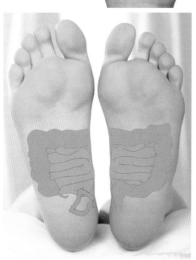

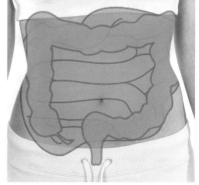

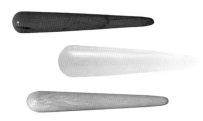

Red Jasper, Rose Quartz, Fossil Wood

Movement Integration

The third large system is the motoric system of the body. This corresponds to a particular density of information. Well-known scientists depart from the premise that our upright posture, and the sophisticated development of our hands connected with it, were the prerequisites for our intellectual faculties. But, to explore this further, let us just take the simple example from everyday life of carrying a cup of coffee up stairs. Several internally attuned processes are at work, all at the same time; molecules activate the cells of the muscles via nerve impulses, movement programmes regulate the orderly sequence of tensions in the individual muscles, and they, in turn, are attuned to the perceptions of our senses. If all this were not taking place, we would fail at the very next manoeuvre with the cup while negotiating our 'obstacle course'. Our motoric system, however, is able to master this, and the multitude of other daily challenges, without our having to think about it, and nearly always successfully.

In crystal healing, whenever we want to emphasize the fact that the qualities of crystals are very difficult to grasp with the intellect, we can use these physical communication processes as an example for how we may imagine the influences of the crystal wands. They support the motoric activity programme on the level of the 'mechanistic language' of the body, and thus help improve our inner balance and make our movement processes more fluid.

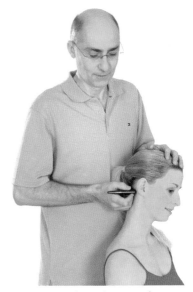

Crystal Wand Massage for Movement Coordination

The most important crystal wand for movement coordination is Bloodstone, although from the great variety available you can source suitable crystals wands made of Amethyst, Magnesite, Obsidian, or other suitable crystal qualities as described in the portraits (pages 22-39).

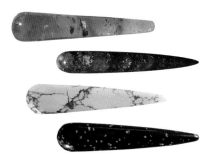

Amethyst, Bloodstone, Magnesite, Obsidian

Massage for Movement Integration

Our spines contain the data motorway for all movement impulses. Thus the tuning described on page 83 is also the basic treatment for optimizing the motoric system. Use a different crystal wand in this case though, one that is in keeping with the aim of the treatment. Afterwards gently massage, stroking first the back of the legs towards the feet and then the arms down to the hands, about 3 to 4 times with the crystal wand. When massaging the legs, follow the middle line in each case from the buttocks down to the soles of the feet; with the arms, go from the shoulder to the backs of the hands. Therapists who have experience with acupressure may follow the meridian lines.

Whether to use the pointed or rounded end of the crystal can best be decided through a brief test. Should any problem points emerge, they can be balanced with the basic unblocking procedure.

For a shorter massage treatment, finish with stroking lines along the spine, and then allow the client to rest afterwards, covered up, for a little while.

If it is to be a more comprehensive or extended treatment, continue the crystal wand massage on the client's front.

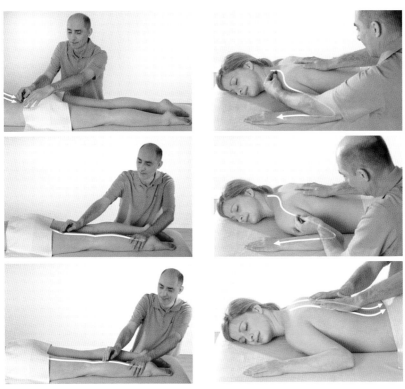

Massage for Integrating Movement (Short Treatment)

In addition to the performing of basic unblocking procedures, the gentle stroking movements of the massage can be interrupted in favour of pleasant circling at and around the joints, if it feels appropriate to do so. These circular massage movements have also proven to be an excellent daily self-help treatment for the joints, and can be carried out through clothing.

The next treatment element, massage of the head, can also be done on its own, and is a wonderfully enriching practice to include in a course on head massage, especially for hairdressers. Using small, gentle, circular movements, we massage the four strips that were discovered about 30 years ago by the Austrian doctor, Hans Zeitler, in the course of skull acupuncture. Beginning

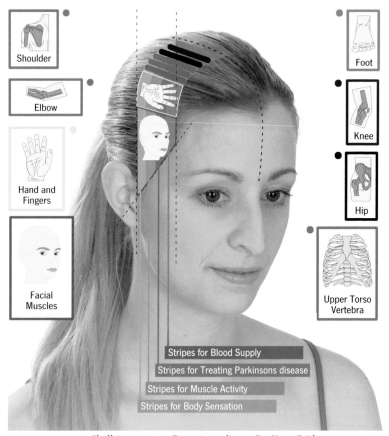

Skull Acupuncture Zones According to Dr. Hans Zeitler

from the middle of the head, we first carry out the little circular movements of treatment along the right side of the head and, after massaging those four strips, we work on the left side of the head in the same manner.

To finish the massage, perform light finger movements along the line of the neck, starting in the middle and moving left and right, at the same time, stroking outwards about 3-5 times. Then allow the client to rest, covered up, for a few minutes.

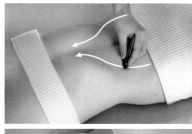

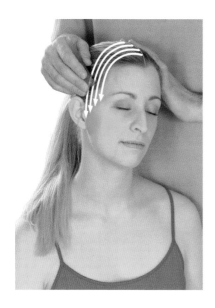

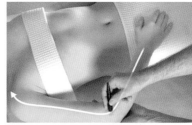

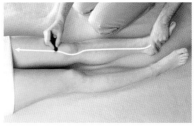

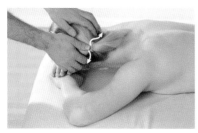

Massage for Movement Integration
(Extended Treatment)

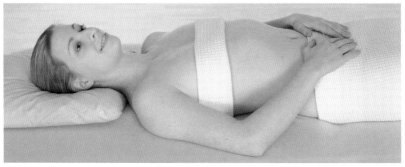

The Relaxation Programme

Becoming tense and letting go are factors that determine our lives – the art consists of finding the right mode in which to operate at any given time. If faced with an interesting challenge, relaxation would not be helpful. However, a romantic candlelit dinner is something we would only be able to enjoy in an inwardly relaxed state.

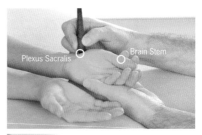

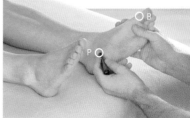

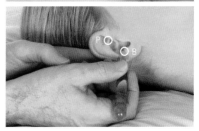

Reflex Zones of the Autonomic Nervous System

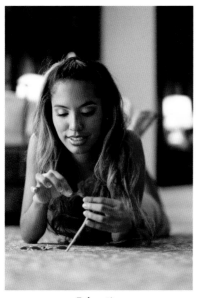

Relaxation

Readiness for action, as well as the need for peace and quiet, are transmitted by the autonomic nervous system. This part of the nervous system, which is absolutely ancient in terms of our evolution, is what we work with during crystal reflex massages to bring the body and soul more serenity; crystals are able to accomplish real miracles when it comes to achieving relaxation in the appropriate zones. The zones in question are those of the brain stem and the nervous system of the belly. The best places to access these reflex zones are through the hands, the feet, the ears and the belly.

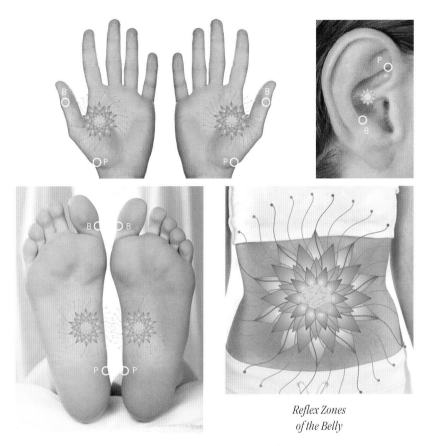

Reflex Zones
of the Belly

The brain stem is situated at the junction of the spinal cord and the brain. In addition to controlling the heart and breathing, there are also important autonomic switching points and nerve nuclei situated there. The importance of our other autonomic system, the nervous system of the belly, was underestimated for a long time. Feeling good comes from the belly. The saying 'butterflies in your belly' indi-

cates this fact, as well as more recent research that discovered an autonomic control centre there that also plays an important role for the immune system. Scientists refer to it as 'GALT' – gut associated lymphoid tissue. The nervous system of the belly, which is connected with the GALT, may be regarded as our 'second brain'. Thus it is important to pay particular attention to the belly area when carrying out reflex massages. In

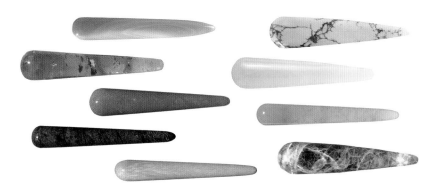

Agate, Amethyst, Aventurine, Dumortierite, Fossil Wood (left, from top),
Magnesite, Rose Quartz, Serpentine, Sodalite (right, from top)

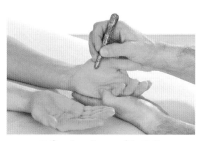

Reflexology Zones of the Belly

addition to one's feeling of wellbeing, the ability to make decisions 'from the gut', so to speak, is also vastly improved. This is an ability we need in all aspects of our lives, not only in our daily work or profession.

From these two autonomic control centres, we are able to bring ourselves down from inner 'high revs' tension back to more normal 'revolutions' - the sort of relaxation associated with a kind of competent composure. The Relax-Quick Programme described below is

excellently suited to self-treatment; however, the enjoyment of the Relax-Pleasure Programme is experienced most fully when we place ourselves in the hands of another, or when we receive this treatment from a professional.

The classic crystal wands for the Relaxation Programme are Aventurine, Amethyst, Magnesite, Sodalite, Agate, Dumortierite, Rose Quartz, Serpentine, Fossil Wood, or other relaxing crystals from the list in the 'Basics' chapter.

The Relax-Quick Programme

This quick programme lasts for no longer than 2-3 minutes, and yet it is powerful enough to bring relief in acutely stressful situations.

Breathe in and out deeply three times, and, for the following three breaths, use a crystal wand from the

Relax Programme on the spinal zones of one hand, from the tip of the thumb to the wrist. The choice of relax-crystal wand will be completely according to intuition. After doing the same to the other hand, carry out basic unblocking at the reflex zones of the brain stem on both hands (one after the other) to ensure that the autonomic nervous system is switched to better functioning.

As a complementary measure, afterwards massage the reflex zones of the belly, working through, point by point, with circling motions in a serpent-like course. The finale will consist of further stroking movements along the spinal zones.

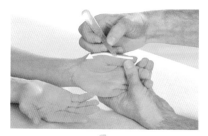

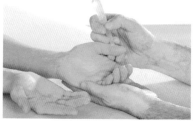

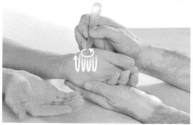

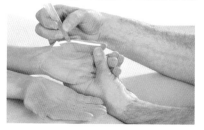

The Relax-Quick Programme

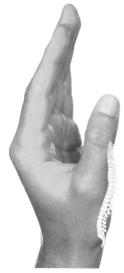

Spinal Column Zone on the Hand

The Relax-Pleasure Programme

When there is more time available, the Relax-Pleasure Programme ensures a deep relaxation experience on all levels. Always begin such a treatment by synchronizing your breathing rhythm to that of your client. For this, the client will be lying comfortably on his or her back; stand or sit beside them and lay one hand on his/her tummy and attune to their breathing rhythm. Throughout the treatment, remember to pay attention to breathing in synchrony.

After synchronizing the breath, test for the best possible crystal wand for this treatment from the assortment of balancing crystals. Using the chosen crystal, carry out stroking motions along the spinal zones and perform basic unblocking of the brain stem reflex zones, just as you would for the Quick-Relax Programme. After that, massage the reflex zones of the small and large intestines with the rounded end of the crystal. These are the zones where we have access to the autonomic abdominal nervous system. Experience has

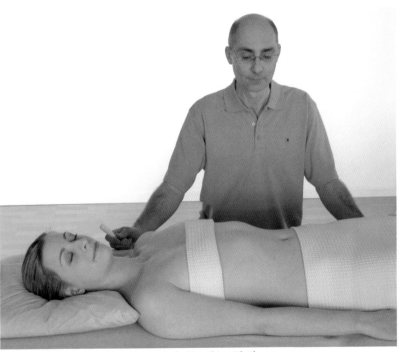

Attune to the Breathing Rhythm

shown that it is helpful to use a few drops of a good massage oil (for example, the crystal oil 'Serenity')* or a pea-size amount of PEKANA crystal balm (for example, No. 3 yellow, or No. 6 dark blue).* The oil or the balm should be spread across your palms and then gently massaged into the client's belly or the referring reflexology zones.

The holds to use for this are mainly slow circling movements in unison with the breathing rhythm of the client. In the course of this lovely massage, which should last about 10–15 minutes, you may carry out a basic unblocking procedure for each of the areas where you detect more tension (please don't exceed more than five basic unblocking procedures per session). During the course of such an abdominal massage the autonomic nervous system is calmed, and you are likely to experience that the client is breathing visibly deeper into the abdominal area.

After that, we may even employ the 'elevator technique' on the front of the body as a professional variation. After briefly carrying out a further 'yes'–'no' calibration, (see pulse test or dowsing test in the 'Basics' chapter), move the crystal wand along the mid-line of the tummy from below upwards (never the other way round, unless this is a love

* see also the 'Basics' chapter.

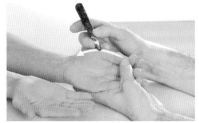

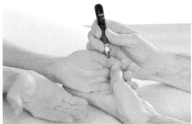

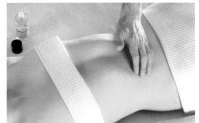

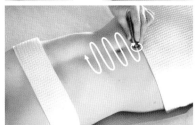

The Relax-Pleasure Programme

massage!), imagining it rising up like an elevator. Stop the elevator when you reach a place where you detect a 'no' signal. Leave the elevator there and follow the imagined course of the ribs

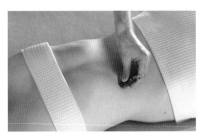

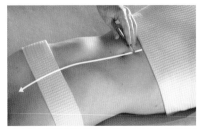

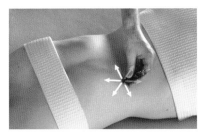

Basic Unblocking of the Leader Zone

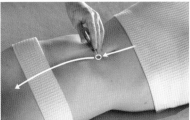

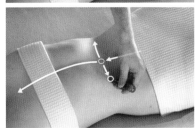

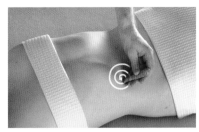

Conducting Away Excess Energy

The Elevator Technique

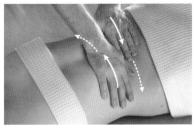

Adding Energy

to the left and then to the right, until you identify another point where a 'no' signal appears. Experience has shown that this is the 'leader zone', via which you can achieve maximum relaxation for the client. For this purpose, first carry out a basic unblocking on this 'leader zone'. After that, test whether this zone requires additional energy or for energy to be conducted away. Should this zone require calming, continue with an appropriate crystal wand

Final Cross-stroking

and conduct the energy away from the point using sunray strokes. If, however, the tests reveal a desire for more energy, then you need to test for a crystal wand for treating this point that will lend more power; use spiral circling motions to conduct energy to the centre of this point. Even if it may initially sound contradictory, it sometimes requires some extra energy for relaxation. The end of the treatment will consist of flat, cross-stroking motions of the hands across the tummy in the rhythm of the client's breathing. After that, allow him/her some time to rest.

Even if calming the waves of emotion and the stream of thoughts is one of the most difficult of tasks, the Relax Programme with crystal wands allows us to switch the autonomic nervous system relatively easily to a mode of relaxation and wellbeing.

The Power Programme

How familiar are you with this scenario? You are supposed to be carrying out some urgent task or making an important phone call, but instead you are playing with your pencil, or dreaming of changing things in your garden, or you are compiling a guest list for your next dinner party. In brief, you lack that igniting spark – at least for the task you are supposed to be accomplishing. Alas, experience has shown that all those lovely substitute targets of our motivation would inevitably fall victim to other dreams were they to be the task at hand.

Naturally, the first question should be whether these random thoughts might be a necessary 'time out' in a turbulent field of diverse challenges and demands, and that our subconscious mind simply sends us into a dream state so that we can replenish our energy. Unfortunately, in such states of exhaustion, or even in momentary states of energy lack, this programme will not

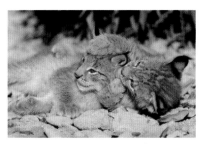

Basic Motive 'Towards'

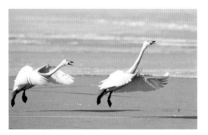

Basic Motive 'Away From'

help. The igniting spark of our motivation can be identified through the autonomic nervous system. Two motives are known; one is the motive 'towards' joy, lust or food – the other is 'away from' danger or reluctance. Experience has shown that crystal reflex massage makes possible highly effective strategies for activating the 'towards' motive, and thus awakens motivation. Crystals play just as important a role in this as the reflex zones, through which we may activate our powers.

And looking deeper, 'activating' means supporting the body and the soul to organize a better access to energy. Two organs in our bodies are essentially responsible for this – the liver and the pancreas. While the liver places nutrients from food at our disposal, the pancreas ensures optimal energy management.

The Instant Power Programme

This programme takes 2–3 minutes.

The 'waking up hold' is about activating the brain zones. First, generously knead each of the fingertips and toe tips. The effect is even more intense if you use a power crystal to playfully work through these zones.

Afterwards, using the same crystal wand, vigorously stroke the spinal zones (for example on the hands and feet, on each side) 5–7 times, starting below from the pelvic zones up to the head zones.

The classic crystal wands for the activation of energy reserves are Red Jasper, Landscape Jasper, Snowflake Obsidian, orange Calcite, and Fossil Wood. In

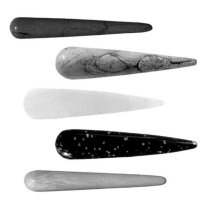

Red Jasper, Landscape Jasper, orange Calcite, Snowflake Obsidian, Fossil Wood

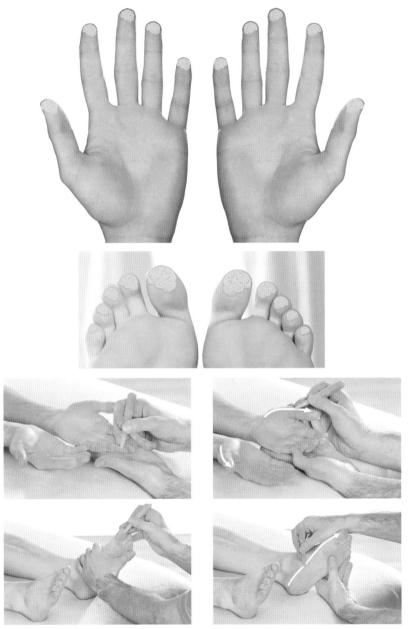

The Instant Power Programme

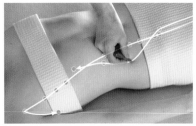

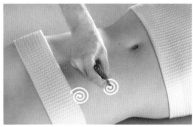

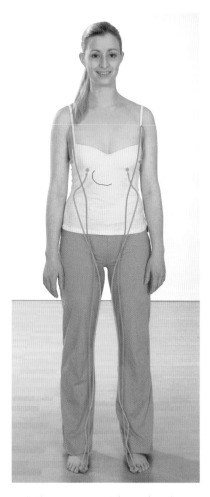

The Comprehensive
Power Programme

addition to these, you can find other suitable crystal wands from the list in the 'Basics' chapter.

To complement this treatment, stroke the meridians* of the liver and the spleen/pancreas about 5-7 times

with the power crystal wand and massage with spiral circling motions any noticeable points along the meridians. Naturally, we are also free, at any time, to check the other meridians and to support the weak meridians using the crystal wand in the direction of the flow.

* Meridians are energy channels in acupuncture and traditional Chinese medicine.

The Direction of Flow of Acupressure Meridians

In acupressure, the energy flows within energy channels in a very specific direction. Traditional Chinese medicine often begins the list of meridians with the lung. These meridians, as well as the energy channels of the heart and the circulation, begin at the chest cavity near the armpits, and flow in the direction of the fingers where they termi-nate. The energies of the meridians of the large intestine, the small intestine and the triple warmer emerge in the fingers, and then flow to the head. That is where the meridians of the stomach, bladder and gall bladder begin, which, in turn, end at the feet. Finally, the feet are where the meridians of the spleen, the liver, and the kidneys begin, which have their terminal points at the chest.

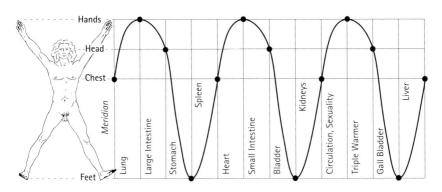

The Beauty Programme

Beauty has many facets and serves many backgrounds, such as personal ideals, cultural values, trends of the times, just to name a few. To witness this, we need only compare our ideas of beauty with those of people in other countries. In spite of all the differences, however, there is still an overall 'biology of beauty', which the magazine 'News-week' once used as the title of an issue; everywhere, all over the world, relaxed faces and people with smooth fluid movements are perceived as beautiful and attractive. This shows once again that beauty comes from an inner atti-tude that affects external appearance.

In order to achieve this external effect, people of all times have employed various methods, including crystals. In addition to their obvious use as jew-ellery, crystals promote inner balance

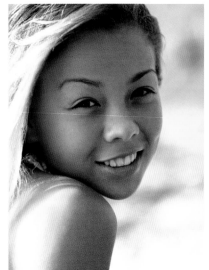
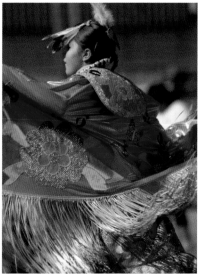

Beauty: Relaxed Faces and Flowing Movements

and thus create beauty. This function is achieved especially by the three classic crystals, Rock Crystal, Amethyst and Rose Quartz. It is hardly surprising then that people usually name these three crystals as the 'best' crystals, immediately after the Diamond.

In beauty treatments, the main application is massage of the face, though of course we must be sure not to neglect the rest of the body, the 'Temple of the Soul'. To choose the crystal wand that will lead in the direction of beauty, just follow your feeling. Those deeper

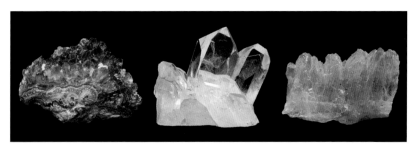

Rock Crystal, Amethyst, and Rose Quartz - Beauty Classics

images of beauty are simply not accessible to the intellect. Once you have chosen a crystal, carry out a pleasant massage and support it with a crystal oil. If you have chosen Rock Crystal, the crystal oil 'Regeneration' is the suitable one. To accompany the Amethyst massage, use 'Composure' or 'Power of Spirit', and with Rose Quartz use 'In the Flow'.*

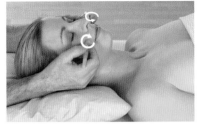

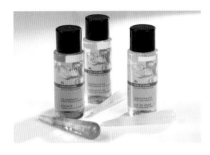

When giving a facial massage of this kind, the most pleasant and best way of proceeding is with two wands of the same crystal. Monika Grundmann describes this in detail in her book, *Crystal Balance*.**

For the facial massage, circle gently and pleasantly over the face with the rounded end of the crystal wand. During the course of the treatment you will, at times, be 'stopped' or 'braked' by the tissue or by your own feeling. If you perceive such a point or zone, balance

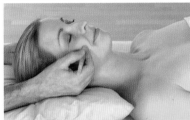

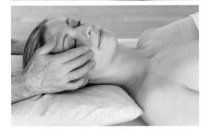

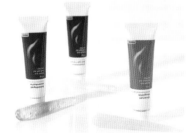

The Beauty Programme

* see also the chapter on 'Basics'
** Monika Grundmann, *Crystal Balance*, Earthdancer a Findhorn Press Imprint, 2008

it with a basic unblocking procedure and afterwards use a PEKANA crystal balm to treat the area. With Rock Crystal use balm No. 5 (medium blue), for

Amethyst use No. 7 (violet), and for Rose Quartz use No. 1 (red). When in doubt, always test for the suitable balm.

For a more comprehensive beauty concept, you could follow the treatment with a movement integration section from the Wellness Programme or from the Love Programme.

The Love Programme

'Love is demonstrated in myriad ways; it has no form or shape, no boundaries, and nothing we could hold onto.'* All of us fill the concept of love with our own, very personal wishes and experiences. Sometimes we are brushed by the wings of fulfilment. Those are moments in which we can feel, in the depths of our souls, that the wish for the other person's happiness is reciprocated.

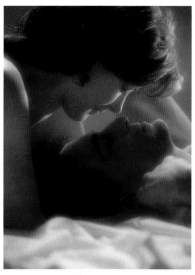

Love, Fulfilment, Happiness

* *A Little Bird*, Words and music by Jerry Jeff Walker, arranged and adapted by Harry Belafonte: 'I said that love takes many shapes: it has no forms, has no boundaries has no grips to hold...'

Amor or Eros stand for powerful elementary forces in Nature, which are expressed through the union of the male and female principles. The most impressive description of this was by Plato, who spoke of the 'spherical being' who had such great powers that even the Olympian gods were challenged by it. When Zeus recognized this danger, he took one of his lightning bolts and divided the spherical being into two halves - into a man and a woman. Ever since then, we have been trying to get back our original power through sexual union. During love massage in particular, we become aware that we can only experience such powers together and never possess them alone.

It is clear that regulation of all love impulses occurs via the heart. Crystal reflex massage gives us an opportunity for touching the person being massaged from our own heart space, thereby reaching out from heart to heart. And we know from crystal healing research that Rose Quartz, Red Aventurine and Serpentine promote the ability to love. As an addition, and to dissolve tension, Serpentine, as well as the 'take it easy' crystal, Dumortierite, are very helpful.

As always, begin with synchronizing your breathing with that of the person being massaged, who is lying in a relaxed position on his/her back.

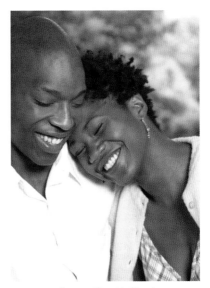

Contact Heart to Heart

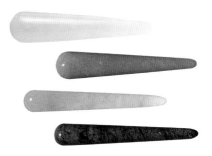

Rose Quartz, Red Aventurine, Serpentine, Dumortierite

Begin the massage by passing the crystal wands a few times (3-5 times) on each side down the arms from the armpit to the palms of the hands. Follow that with stroking movements

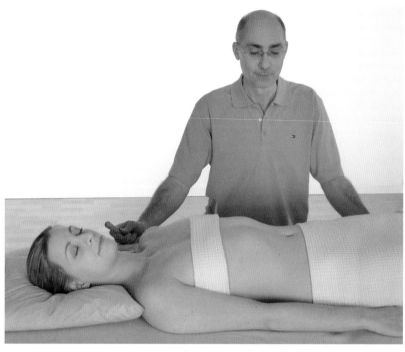

Tune In to the Breathing Rhythm

beginning from the soles of the feet and along the inner edges of the legs up to the groin area.

After that, perform 3–5 strokes along the mid-line from the hollow immediately above the breastbone down to the edge of the pelvic rim. (The Love Programme is the only application in which we stroke from the top downwards on the front side of the torso!) After the massage movements along the mid-line, follow with further strokes on

the left and the right of the mid-line, at intervals of about two finger-widths. Remember to always keep the same breathing rhythm as the person being massaged.

These treatments can be equally enjoyable and deeply moving for both the person being massaged and the person massaging. Beauty unfolds, radiating outwardly. This opening of the heart gives both people the opportunity to experience deep love on a soul level.

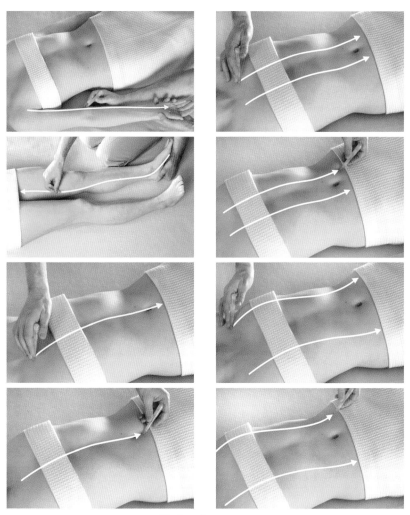

The Love Programme

The Protection Programme

Imagine you have been carrying out your massages with the best possible intentions, only to realize that, along with your positive energies, you have been sending out your personal ideas, fears, anxieties, or even your conflict with your next-door neighbour.

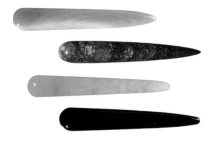

Agate, Bloodstone, Serpentine, Tourmaline Schorl

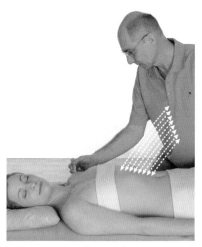

The Transference of Energies

In the worst-case scenario, we pass those energies over to the other person, and, without realizing it, transfer to them our own personality programme. Or the other way round, we may take on energies from the person you are treating. Maybe both. This often happens in treatments if we open ourselves up too much. Then, for a few days afterwards, we may feel as if we are being controlled by outside forces.

Since about 1970, treatments have increasingly taken on an energetic character, or have integrated aspects of an energetic nature. Psychosomatics is no longer rejected as an exotic notion, and many methods that would have been considered 'esoteric' even twenty years ago, have meanwhile become components of recognized non-medical treatments. The necessity for protection from energies is unfortunately often forgotten, even though it is an essential part of any energetic treatment.

Energies are meant to flow, but they are not meant to burden us. In principle, the grounding exercise on page 65 has been tried and tested as a protection against external energies. Beyond that, crystals can be used to purify and filter energies for the purposes of protection. Usually a brief stimulus at the beginning of a treatment will suffice to clear the flow of energies between practitioner and client. Crystal wands made of Agate, Bloodstone, Serpentine and Tourmaline Schorl have proven to be particularly successful.

The protective element at the beginning of a massage treatment can consist of moving a protective crystal wand 1–2 times along the back and spinal zones on the client's hands and feet, and from the neck downward to the sacrum. Thus the energies may flow unhindered during the treatment. Should you have the feeling that there might be 'transmission traces' still present at the end of the massage, you can remove them with the same stroking movements.

With this Protection Programme you will be able to create a stable environment in which to give treatments, a space that is protected and free from energetic turbulence. For further protection, crystal water sprays can be used, or you can set up a protective 'Self-regulating System' of crystals in your treatment room. Michael Gienger describes these beautifully in his little volume, *Purifying Crystals*.* Visualisations can also build up protection. A detailed description of this can be found in the book, *Crystal Massage for Health and Healing.* **

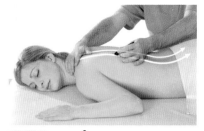
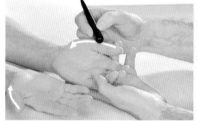
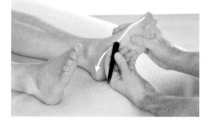

The Protection Programme

* M. Gienger, *Purifying Crystals*, Earthdancer a Findhorn Press Imprint, 2008
** M. Gienger, *Crystal Massage for Health and Healing*, Earthdancer a Findhorn Press Imprint, 2006

A Professional Reflex Zone Massage with Crystal Wands

As described in the *Pschyrembel®* – *Wörterbuch Naturheilkunde [Dictionary of Natural Healing]*, reflex zones are 'areas of the skin and mucous membranes, whose structure, colouring, and other characteristics provide evidence about regulatory disorders in the organs or other body structures and which can also be used for treatment'. Massaging the reflex zones with crystal wands, however, is more than just connecting up two methods. It is the synthesis of two ancient principles of treatment that complement each other energetically. Crystals play a central role in many ancient myths and legends, which suggests that people were harnessing the effects of crystals long before writing was invented. Greek and Roman authors, such as Theophrastus, Dioskurides and Pliny, as well as medieval scholars such as Hildegard von Bingen,* then later recorded crystal applications in writing.

The understanding of reflex zones also dates back to humankind's 'childhood'. The first documented evidence for knowledge of reflex zones is the

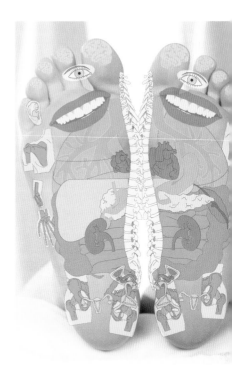

5,300 year-old tattoo on the back of 'Ötzi', a male body found frozen in ice in the Alps, that depicts a system surprisingly similar to acupuncture. Australian and African Bushmen, whose social forms are probably closest to those of the Stone Age, also use body painting and tattooing in rituals for health. If we look at the timeline of humankind, reflex zone treatment had already been carried out in Central Europe for 1,000 years before the Egyptians depicted reflex zone massage of the hands and feet in a physician's tomb in Sakkara

* Michael Gienger, *Die Heilsteine der Hildegard von Bingen*, Neue Erde, Saarbrücken, 2004

around 2,300BC. This fact about the history of medical science is still rarely honoured or appreciated.

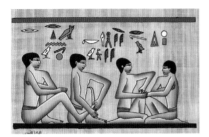

Crystals, as well as reflex zones, work in ways that are often inexplicable. Both were first employed purely intuitively, then magically, and now increasingly systematically, for healing purposes. With a few exceptions, it has hitherto never been possible to present a model for explaining how crystals and reflex zones work, in what way an impulse arrives at a disturbed organ, or how these impulses find exactly those zones or principles that relate to a specific organ. Naturally, we are judging based on the criteria that our current scientific community recognizes as valid. The reflex zones on the back alone, which are assigned to the different levels of the spine, were explained by Henry Head in 1893. But even then, it took 30 years before an appropriate means of treatment was established through the physiotherapist, Elizabeth Diecke, in 1929, which took the form of connective tissue massage. Ms. Diecke was suffering from an arterial blockage disease of the legs in 1928 and had already booked an appointment for an amputation, when she began, by chance, to move her fingers in a 'plough-like' fashion along the skin of her lower back. This caused her to feel a curious tingling sensation in her legs. Through

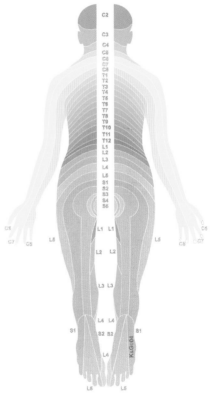

'Dermatoms' or 'Head's Zones'
on the Back

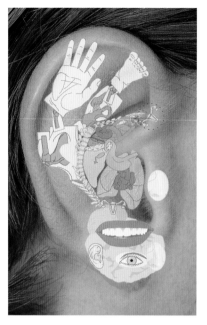

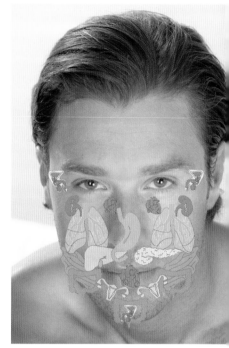

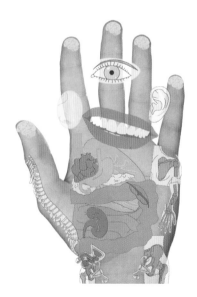

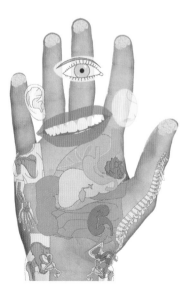

consistent self-massage she was finally able to avoid the loss of her leg, and went on to develop this form of treatment.

In addition to the reflex zones on the back, we know of about 30 further reflex zone systems on the surfaces of our bodies. The best known of these are on the hands and feet. But reflex zones can also be found on the skull, the face, and the ears, and we may rightly refer to them as the maps of our state of health.

My own personal path to the reflex zones began through my training as a masseur using connective tissue massage. The reactions that a few finger movements could trigger in the subcutaneous connective tissue were simply fascinating. People were able to breathe better and more deeply, back problems disappeared, bladder problems were improved and the intestines began to work properly again. However, the effects can also be quite drastic. For example, the intestines may react with diarrhoea or the circulation may become temporarily weaker. Even headaches may occur for a short while. Usually these reactions disappear again after a few minutes rest. Later I was to discover that extreme reactions like these can also occur when using crystals.

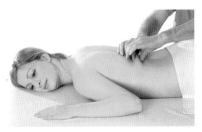

Connective Tissue Massage on the Back

The more I learned about handling crystals and the reflex zones, the clearer it became that both are connected with the organisation of our energy field and the streams of energy that affect us. This was the junction point between crystals and reflex zones for which I had been searching for so long. Unfortunately, when I first started using them in combination, the results were not particularly convincing. People did not react in ways I had expected. I became impatient, and felt that I was somehow not approaching the subject in the right way.

Thus began a period of much experimentation. I enjoyed a lot of support from the Marco Schreier team and from Walter von Holst. Finally it was Marco Schreier who took up my suggestion to polish suitable minerals into the shape of wands. As I had for a long time been using wands made of wood as a supportive aid when giving massages, I was overjoyed that this shape could now be realized in the form of crystal wands.

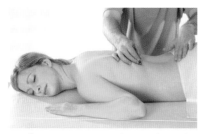

Reflex Zone Massage with Crystal Wands

Kinesiological tests, as well as my father's pendulum, confirmed that we were on the right track. The thicker end was polished to a rounded shape, while the other end terminated in a gentle point – the best shape for reflex zone massage. This meant that I was able to take the burden off my fingers when massaging reflex zones, and of course a crystal wand is always a wonderful tool for other kinds of massage as well. Massage movements that work over larger surface areas of the body can be supported by the larger, rounded end of the crystal, and the pointed end is ideal for targeted stimulation of specific points and for meridian massage.

The first available crystal wands were made of Amethyst, Aventurine, Rock Crystal, Brecciated Jasper, Dalmatian Jasper, Dumortierite, Fluorite, red Jasper, Landscape Jasper, Picasso Marble, Rose Quartz, Lapis Lazuli, and Snowflake Obsidian. We now have some 70 or more crystal wands available.

In spite of everything, I still had not discovered how I could properly awaken the sleeping energies of the crystal wands. Two principles had, however, been confirmed on many occasions: the rounded end of the crystal draws energies from the tissues, and the tip conducts energy in. This was most clearly noticeable with wands made of Rock Crystal. The treatments with Rock Crystal provided amazing relief from hip problems, headaches, and menstrual discomfort. All of this was achieved simply through massage of the appropriate zones in the hand and feet reflex zones using the broad, rounded end. A good friend, alas, had to pay for the gaining of this knowledge when I massaged him using the tip of an Amethyst wand, which resulting in an increase in symptoms in the shoulder zone. With time it became ever clearer that acute conditions with an excess of energy require massage with the thick end of the wand of a balancing crystal, and chronic con-

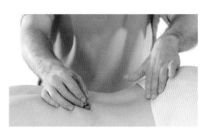

*Connective Tissue Massage
with a Crystal Wand*

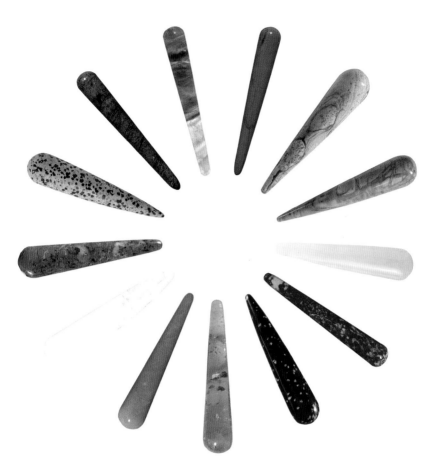

Clockwise from bottom centre: Amethyst, Aventurine, Rock Crystal, Brecciated Jasper, Dalmatian Jasper, Dumortierite, Fluorite, red Jasper, Landscape Jasper, Picasso Marble, Rose Quartz, Lapis Lazuli, Snowflake Obsidian

ditions with a lack of energy require massage with the tip of activating crystals. However, it was still unclear to me how I could draw in the qualities of the crystals for use with reflex zones. In contrast to the effects of the 'laying on' of crystals, the qualities of the crystals did not seem to come through properly in a relatively short reflex zone massage, and any effects could probably be explained by the use of the reflex zones alone – not by the quality of the crystal.

All these doubts were answered through experience. For instance, a foot reflex zone massage balanced the intestine and digestion, although I had not paid special attention to those reflex zones. But brown Landscape Jasper, which I had used for the massage, is clearly applicable to this organ system in its effects.

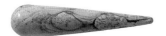

Crystal Wands Made of Landscape Jasper

On another occasion I passed a wand made of red Jasper very lightly over the neck and head zones. My client suddenly developed a headache. As soon as I swapped the Jasper for an Aventurine wand, the situation was defused and the pain immediately disappeared.

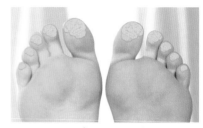

Brain Reflex Zones on the Feet

The last doubts were swept away through an experience with a client who had arrived at my practise with a bladder infection and cold feet. We know of a zone among the skull reflex zones that never fails to warm cold from the inside, within minutes.

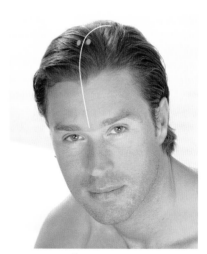

Foot Reflex Zones on the Head

Imagine how astonished I was when I massaged this zone and there was no reaction! I had picked up a crystal that

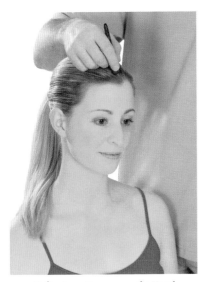

*Reflex Zone Massage on the Head
for Warm Feet*

time. With the expansion of my selection of crystal wands and the frequent changing, it became clear to me that I needed a different way of proceeding, a quieter method of treatment. Many experiences and conversations later, I came to the conclusion that in reflex zone massage with crystal wands the important thing is to identify and treat the 'leader zone'. This is the reflex zone that indicates the overall theme and can resolve the issue. As soon as that reflex zone is unblocked, the other zones simply follow, like the domino effect.

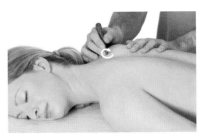

Massage of the Gall Bladder Zone

happened to be at arm's reach, a Picasso Marble. Surprised by this failure, I changed the crystal and intuitively took the 'classic' for cold extremities, a Snowflake Obsidian. Within seconds the client experienced prickling and streaming sensations in the feet, and finally convinced me that the connection between crystal wands and reflex zones constituted an extremely useful combination.

In the beginning I changed crystal wands quite frequently during a reflex zone treatment. Whenever it emerged that a different organ system was unbalanced, a different wand would be employed, testing for the right one each

For example, if there is a weakness in the digestive processes, there could be several possible causes. One of them might be a weakened functioning of the gall bladder; another might be a stomach problem; and naturally, the intestine might be ailing. Only in the third case would the theme be removed through massage of the intestine zones. With the other causes, we would only achieve a short-term alleviation of the symptoms. This is true also for the energetic level. A weak gall bladder function connected with lack of drive, or lack of a healthy aggression response, requires massage of the gall bladder zones with red Jasper. If we used a Landscape Jasper instead, the classic 'intestine crystal', we would be employing an unsuitable energetic principle and success would be questionable. Once the leader principle is found, such disturbances are easier to resolve. The trick is to locate the leader zone! Luckily, the existence of the reflex zones makes possible a simple search for the principle and the zone from which a problem has started.

How to Find the Leader Zone

A certain technique has emerged for the search for the leader zone, a method that has been tried and tested for reflex zone massage. The tests described here use the pulse quality and breathing frequency, but testing can be carried out equally well using a pendulum, a dowsing rod, or a kinesiological muscle test.

Choose a crystal wand made of Rock Crystal, Chalcedony, or a suitable crystal wand with neutral quality from the list in the 'Basics' chapter, and then stroke with a light touch along the spinal reflex zone from below upward (see illustration).

At the same time, and with your other hand, test the pulse at the wrist or at the carotid artery (carefully!!). While moving the wand upwards, pay attention to the quality of the pulse. At those points where the pulse rate clearly changes, stop briefly and make a mental

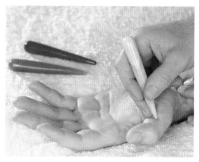

Identifying a Change in the Pulse Rate

note of the location. Then carry on. It is insignificant whether the pulse is stronger or weaker, slower or faster, tenser or broader, harder or softer, whether it pounds, is thread-like, flowing, or becomes less emphatic. The crucial thing is the intensity of the change. In this way, you will obtain one to three different locations.

120

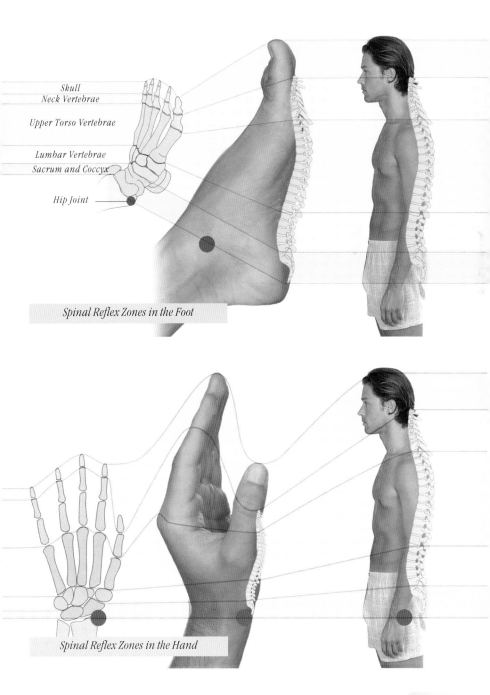

Skull
Neck Vertebrae

Upper Torso Vertebrae

Lumbar Vertebrae
Sacrum and Coccyx

Hip Joint

Spinal Reflex Zones in the Foot

Spinal Reflex Zones in the Hand

Now repeat the procedure; this time concentrate on sensing the most intense signal. If you are still undecided, simply repeat again.

The point you have now identified in the spinal zone indicates the way to the leader zone. Using this departure point, move with the broad end of the wand gently through the reflex zones of the spinal level in question. You are then checking, so to speak, the 'corridor' from which this level is supplied.

Pay special attention to the client's breathing. Notice that your client demonstrates different reactions in his/her breathing. At the point where the breath becomes shorter or even stops, you will have found the leader reflex zone. If you check at this point with your fingers, you will sense that this zone feels somehow different to the surrounding area. Therapists can then kinesiologically muscle test the connected organ. This is not necessary in massages intended purely for pleasure; it will suffice to find the suitable crystal wand to unblock the leader zone and then begin the massage.

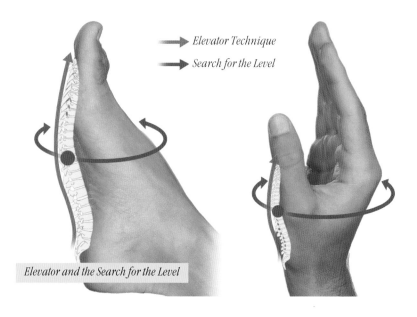

Elevator Technique
Search for the Level
Elevator and the Search for the Level

How to Choose a Crystal Wand

In the case of an impaired reflex zone, there is a fundamental question to ask: 'Does it require balancing, activating, or should the treatment be neutral?' In order to find out, first pick up a neutral crystal – a Rock Crystal, Chalcedony or Snow Quartz, and use it to touch the leader zone. Pay attention to your client's breathing for the duration of four to five breaths. If the breathing becomes longer, deeper or calmer, it is the right choice of crystal. You can stick with that crystal and later on carry out the massage with it. If the breathing becomes less calm or remains un-changed, use the same method to locate the leader zone with a balancing crystal wand, such as Aventurine, Serpentine, or Sodalite. Once again pay attention, for four to five breaths, to the breathing rhythm of your client. If there is again no confirming reaction through deeper, quieter breathing, then repeat the pro-cedure a third time with an activating crystal wand, such as Basalt, Obsidian or red Jasper. The crystal will be the right one when the client's breathing becomes deeper and quieter – even when stimulation is applied. Even if the reaction becomes weaker after a few changes, the test can still be carried out as often as needed.

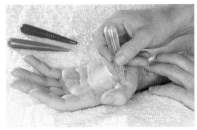

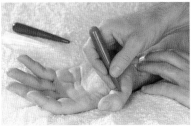

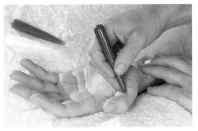

Testing for the Right Crystal Wand

Generally speaking, three crystal wands are enough begin with. Rock Crystal as a neutral crystal, Aventurine for calming, and red Jasper for activat-ing. Experienced masseurs may wish to expand their selection; in the 'Basics' chapter, you will find the crystal wands divided into 'neutral', 'balancing' and 'activating' categories. If you have a good grounding in crystal healing, you may naturally test suitable healing crystals for a targeted therapeutic application. An orientation regarding the effects of the different crystal wands can also be found in the 'Basics' chapter.

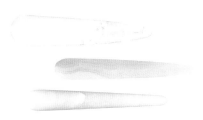

Neutral Wands:
Rock Crystal, Chalcedony, Snow Quartz

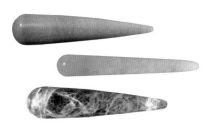

Balancing Crystals:
Aventurine, Serpentine, Sodalite

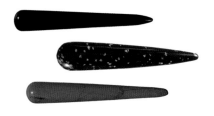

Activating Wands:
Basalt, Obsidian, red Jasper

How to Unblock the Reflex Zones

Once we have a suitable crystal wand, we are almost right in the middle of the massage process. But first, the leader zone requires a basic unblocking. For this basic unblocking, use the crystal wand to remain in the leader zone with gentle pressure, i.e. without moving – for as long as it takes (usually about 1-3 minutes), until your client is breathing deeply. Often this will even be accompanied by a deep sigh. You will notice, at the same time, that the crystal almost 'sinks in'. These are indications that you have removed the interference from the leader zone. Now massage the remaining reflex zones with pleasurable, long, stroking and circling movements.

In order to experience the difference unblocking can make, try doing a reflex zone massage without a basic unblocking of the leader zone, and afterwards a massage with the basic unblocking procedure. This little test has, so far, convinced all concerned.

Should any other reflex zone signal a problem during the massage, carry out a basic unblocking procedure there too. As before, remain quietly in position with your crystal wand and wait for the breathing and tissue relaxation signs in the person you are treating. Depending on the reflex zone system

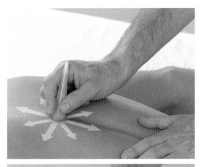

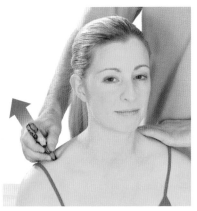

Reduce the intensity if an unpleasant reaction is perceived!

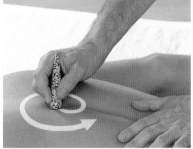

Stroking and Circling

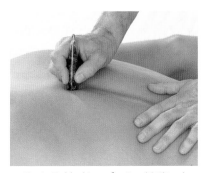

Basic Unblocking after Ewald Kliegel

the back and foot reflex zones. With these massages, always be sure that all holds and applications are thoroughly pleasurable and lend a sense of well-being. If, despite your best efforts, an impulse is perceived as unpleasant or even painful, the intensity should be reduced to the point that the touch or the massage hold feels good again (for you AND your client).

addressed and the theme of the massage, a full massage in this form can take from three minutes (for example, as a fast treatment on the hands) up to an hour with an extensive massage of

To finish a reflex zone treatment, the entire reflex zone system – the back, the hands and the feet – can be massaged again thoroughly with the hands. After that, allow the client to rest for a little while. When giving such a massage to a friend or partner, it has been shown that a reciprocal treatment should not be undertaken immediately afterwards. It is much better to reserve an evening or a session exclusively for one massage

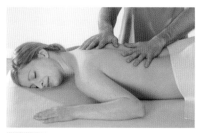

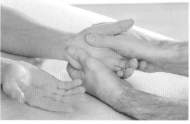

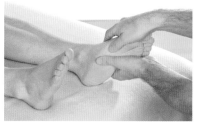

For a finale, give an
extensive massage by hand!

and then to enjoy the other one on a different day. In this way, you and your friend or partner will get the most out of the massages.

How the Energies Take Effect

Even with such a simple technique, there are deep-reaching effects. In order to deepen your understanding still further, I would now like to take you on a little trip into the basics of reflex zones.

If we observe the physical-neurological circumstances in the body, we see that every organ is connected up with the spine. There, information is passed on to the appropriate levels, which is where the control centres for the path to the brain are situated; from there the steering signals go out to the skin in the back reflex zones, and it is from there that the messages from the skin are sent to the organs. In brief, the spine is our energetic central line, our 'data motorway', and the 'elevator' for many types of messages. In principle, within all this information, disturbances are given a priority. For example, if intestinal function is impeded, the regulatory centres are alerted and certain reactions begin in the associated back reflex zones; there, the subcutaneous connective tissue swells a little, skin tension is altered slightly in the zone in question and, via

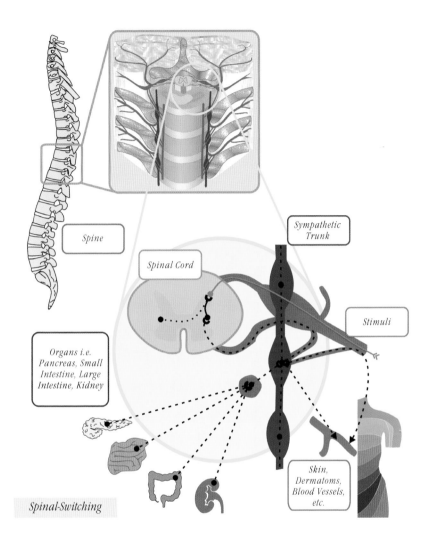

Spine

Sympathetic Trunk

Spinal Cord

Stimuli

Organs i.e. Pancreas, Small Intestine, Large Intestine, Kidney

Skin, Dermatoms, Blood Vessels, etc.

Spinal-Switching

localized heightened blood circulation, a slight reddening of the skin occurs. On the back and the side of the chest these indicators can be explained through neurological switching in the spinal segment in question. In all the other reflex zones this model does not apply, which is clearly demonstrated with the example of the right kidney. This kidney has an identifiable direct nerve-line to its zones on the back, which, in turn, has a switching point in the spine.

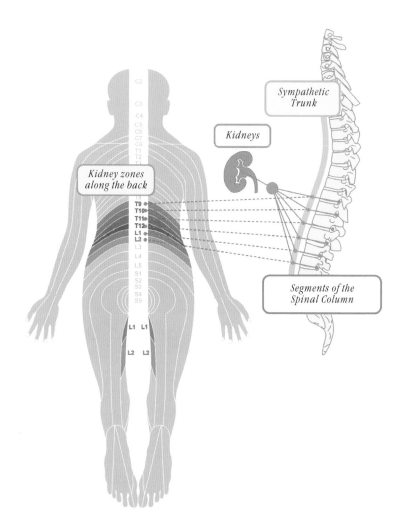

Kidney zones along the back

Sympathetic Trunk

Kidneys

Segments of the Spinal Column

However, a nerve-line such as this does not exist from the kidney to its reflex zones on the feet, the hands, the ears or the face. Nevertheless, it is precisely the reflex zone on the feet that has been confirmed by a scientific study undertaken by the University of Innsbruck in 1999. We should always remember that the reflex zones, which Henry Head discovered in the nineteenth century, marked the beginnings of the science of neurology. This was also the time when electricity and its uses were discovered. That is consequently why electro-mechanical models were used to explain the workings of the back reflex zones, complete with concepts of 'cables' and 'relay stations', all of which was considered to be highly up-to-date and accurate at the time. These explanations are, however, no longer adequate as explanations for the workings of the reflex zones. In order to approach the phenomenon of reflex zones and healing crystals more closely, we have to re-think. Our latest models should be based on the facts of modern, basic science, and in particular on the bio-photon research undertaken by Popp (et al), as well as on modern information transmissions in network systems. We will also have to face the possibility that later generations will smile about our explanations in the same way we do about some of the representatives of the medical sciences who are still clinging to old electro-mechanical thought models.

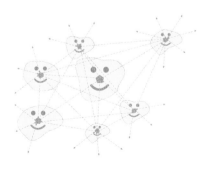

From the 1970s onwards, at the very latest, through research by F. A. Popp we were given confirmation that the human being possesses an energy field, and that acupuncture points and meridians are denser 'areas' within that field. Beyond that, Popp was able to provide evidence that all our cells communicate with each other by means of ultra-weak laser light, as if in a gigantic mobile radio network. Our cells receive a hitherto unknown plethora of information via these communications. If we use this radio network as a basic model, then both the organs, as well as the reflex zones, possess e-mail addresses. In this way, a right kidney that is experiencing a disturbance can pass on a message about the disturbance to the skin, and the reflex zones will send back the relevant treatment stimulations to the kidney. At the target location in question, the information is converted in the form of skin, tissue or organ reactions. At the same time, in the same way, superordinated regulation centres are informed, which, in turn, set in motion autonomic switching of the entire internal environment of that person and also influence his/her psychological state. In our modern network technology, a command given by a computer in Munich can simply activate a printer in Hongkong, and we can

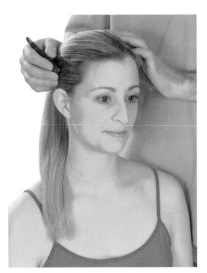

The Crystal as a Frequency Amplifier

assume that our organism with its more than 50 billion cells clearly functions more efficiently than our technological achievements.

In this model we can imagine crystals as frequency amplifiers that support certain energies and dampen others, placing additional information at the disposal of the system and passing on the filtered energies of the therapist.

Whether these models are, in the end, tenable, must remain open at present. The Bible says, 'You may know them by their actions!' and this applies equally to the treatment of reflex zones with crystal wands. The fact remains that reflex zones and crystals work, even if we cannot explain everything. Millions of treatments worldwide have proven it, and the entire history of mankind provides clear evidence in support of it. We are the ones who are continuing to write this history through our daily treatment sessions. Please contribute too. Write that history with us, and begin today with perhaps your very first reflex zone massage with crystal wands.

Addendum

In our efforts to look closely at how we achieve good health, this little story from China* may help us:

'According to an old story, a lord of ancient China once asked his physician, a member of a family of healers, which of them was the most skilled in the art.

The physician, whose reputation was such that his name became synonymous with medical science in China, replied, 'My eldest brother sees the spirit of sickness and removes it before it takes shape, so his name does not get out of the house.

"My eldest brother cures sickness when it is still extremely minute, so his name does not get out of the neighborhood.

"As for me, I puncture veins, prescribe potions, and massage skin, so from time to time my name gets out and is heard among the lords.'"

Chinese physicians and healers of that time were looked after by the village community only if they managed to keep the people healthy. Their art essentially consisted of preventing illnesses. Basically, all treatments should follow this goal. Remaining healthy, in this sense, means consistently moving the internal balance in the direction of good health. Or, put another way, this could be seen as a learning process through which we are becoming more and more competent with the internal tuning of the body and the soul.

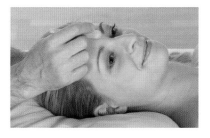

Massage with crystal wands offers a whole spectrum of application possibilities, ranging from improved wellbeing via energetic massage, through to therapy. All of these applications serve good health, which is more than simply the absence of illness. Attempts at holistic good health should not begin when lab results show that things are getting out of hand, or when X-rays demonstrate a change. The best definition of good health was given to us by Hans-Georg Gadamer* when he said, 'Good health is the pleasurable silence of the organs'. But it is also not only a matter of

* As told by Thomas Cleary in the 'Translator's Introduction' to *The Art of War*, Shambhala, Boston, 1988.

* Hans-Georg Gadamer, *Über die Verborgenheit der Gesundheit*, Suhrkamp, Frankfurt, 1993

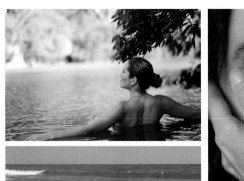

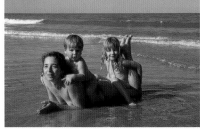

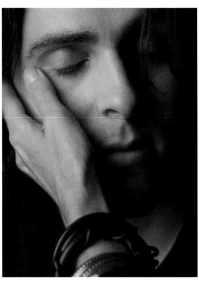

Good Health, Feeling Good, Compassionate Companionship

healthy organs being allowed to be silent – we need to feel good too! Good health has to be extended to incorporate more than just the medical science definition. What were once considered programmes of natural healing are now achieving broader application possibilities through the wellness movement. Whether for healing or wellbeing, the coherence of our energies is involved, and for this, crystals are messengers of the first order and massage simply opens the gates to them.

Actions must follow knowledge and intentions. With this in mind, I would like to encourage you to undertake two things: I would like to invite you to get to know your skin better as the boundary layer and venue for all the measures you undertake. If you then proceed to define the boundaries, you will discover that (adapted freely from Bettina Hesse) no boundaries actually exist in the world of skin perception, merely neighbouring countries. These are good health, feeling good, and compassionate companionship.*

* 'In the kingdom of the senses there are no boundaries, except neighbouring countries – they are called love and pornography'. Bettina Hesse, *Von Sinnen. Ein erotisches Lesebuch*. [Taking Leave of One's Senses - An Erotic Reader], Rowohlt TB Verlag (rororo 23037), Reinbek, 2001

The second request concerns the mineral fruits of the Earth, the crystals. As children we played with pebbles and hoarded colourful stones in our pockets. With increasing age this became 'childish'. I would like to encourage you to retrace those childhood paths. You will discover that your childhood perceptions of the nature of crystals possess serious and real foundations. Naturally, I am hoping that those 'paths' may become well-tended pathways once again...

Whether or not you fulfil these requests, whether you go on to give wellness treatments with crystal wands, employ the wands for energetic massages, or use them for therapies – I wish you much enjoyment and pleasure, and I would be glad to act as your guide with advice and action.

Ewald Kliegel

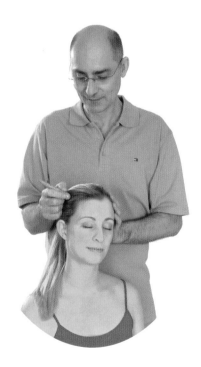

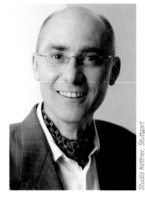

Studio Kettner, Stuttgart

The Author

Ewald Kliegel was born in the country-side of Bavaria (Germany) in 1957, under the sign of Gemini. By the age of 19 he had already heard, and been challenged by, his calling to be a healer and a teacher. His initial contact with healing came about through a practical training in a hospital, which led to his becoming a practicing massage thera-pist and naturopath. Ewald's teaching career began with a practice in a school for handicapped children, which led to

his becoming a lecturer in holistic therapies, reflexology, and gemstone applications. These activities were accompanied by extensive travelling throughout Asia, the establishment of fitness spas in Swiss first-class hotels, and a clinic project at the Cape of Good Hope in South Africa. Everywhere he went Ewald found new approaches to healing, which he then integrated into his work.

Publications:

A number of German publications on various areas of natural healing thera-pies.'

Ewald Kliegel: 'For me the central message of reflexology zones is that they represent the most fascinating phenomena about our skin. Reflexology zones are the "maps of our health". This theme is one that runs through all my publications, and I wish to point out that the surface of our skin contains a veritable "El Dorado" of potential and possibilities, of which we have only understood a mere fraction.'

Contact:
Ewald Kliegel
Rotenbergstrasse 154
D-70190 Stuttgart
info@reflex-international.eu
www.reflex-international.eu

Thanks

Writing is a process that starts with the author's irresistible urge to make his or her own experience accessible to as many interested people as possible, to enthuse them, and to present information that is both interesting and immediately useful. The fact that Andreas Lentz of Neue Erde gave the green light for this book has been a great honour for me, and I am filled with joy and gratitude that the project has succeeded with a veritable concert orchestra of energies. The conductor in the working orchestra, Michael Gienger, was not only a co-initiator of the crystal wand projects, he also provided the introductions to this grandiose undertaking and also contributed in many different ways. Whether in the management of the illustrations, in an editorial capacity, or where suggestions for improvements were concerned, he always hit the right note. In addition, the descriptions of the qualities of crystals came from his pen.

With respect to the crystals, the following contributors should be named, in addition to Michael Gienger: Marco Schreier with his team in Ludwigsburg was willing, more than a decade ago, to polish crystals into the shape of wands and to keep them in stock even during quiet periods. Sabine Schneider-Kuehnle, in particular, was a saving angel during a few explosive stages of development. The Diederichs family in Frauenberg also worked hard to expand the selection of types of crystals and to provide the large range available today. They did not shy away from efforts to make available certain rare types of crystals. Both Walter von Holst and Kerstin Wagner in Stuttgart helped me with excellent consultations on the crystals, and Monika Grundmann gave me good feedback. In particular, it was Monika Grundmann with her Crystal Balance® concept whom I have to thank for the fact that the wands have now achieved extensive application in wellness, cosmetics and therapies.

Ines Blersch supplied us with the wonderful photographic contributions. I was especially impressed with the input of Anja Birkholz who, as the model, would still radiate a fresh and natural quality, even after an eight-hour storm of flash photography. The entire work was then taken by Fred Hageneder and magically transformed into a very accomplished layout. As with all my previous books, my dear friend Thomas Gutsche gave me lots of his time to keep the computer and Internet access running – and this in spite of his demanding job and his family commitments.

Gina Feder and Alexander Zentgraf at their Galeria & Cantina in Murnau chose a special task, as they were sometimes the only ones able to convince me, through liberal doses of art and good red wine, that not everything that was circling around inside my head really needed to be put on paper.

I also had much generous support during the entire writing process from my brother and my sister.

Thank you, all of you!

Literature

Crystal Massage

Michael Gienger, *Crystal Massage for Health and Healing,* Earthdancer a Findhorn Press Imprint, 2006

Monika Grundmann, *Crystal Balance,* Earthdancer a Findhorn Press Imprint, 2008

Crystal Healing

Michael Gienger, *Crystal Power, Crystal Healing*, Cassell/Blandford, 1998

Michael Gienger, *Healing Crystals*, Earthdancer a Findhorn Press Imprint, 2005

Michael Gienger, *The Healing Crystal First Aid Manual*, Earthdancer a Findhorn Press Imprint, 2006

Michael Gienger, *Purifying Crystals*, Earthdancer a Findhorn Press Imprint, 2008

Michael Gienger, Joachim Goebel, *Gem Water*, Earthdancer a Findhorn Press Imprint, 2008

Picture Credits

Ines Blersch, Stuttgart: all photographs except those mentioned below.

Atelier Bunter Hund, Zürich: page 20
Dragon Design: pages 84, 121, 123
Ewald Kliegel, Stuttgart: pages 12, 82, 90, 93, 112-114, 127-129

Barbara Newerla, Rottenburg: page 63
www.photos.com: pages 62 right, 63 top, 79 top, 80, 92, 99, 100 top, 104 top, 106, 107 top, 132.

Sources

Crystal Wands

Crystal wands can be obtained individually or as sets from wellness- or mineral trading companies, or from the author (see www.reflex-international.eu).

Crystal Massage Oils

Monika Grundmann
Cosmetics – crystals – seminars
D-91580 Heilsbronn, Germany
Tel: +49 (0)9872-2999
Fax: +49 (0)9872-2606
info@edelstein-balance.de
www.crystal-balance.com

US and Canada distributor:
www.naturaleurope.com

all other countries:
www.crystal-balance.com

Crystal Balms

PEKANA® Naturheilmittel GmbH
Raiffeisenstrasse 15
D-88353 Kisslegg, Germany
Tel: +49 (0)7563-91160
Fax: +49 (0)7563-2862
info@pekana.com
www.pekana.com

R A Holding DO Regist. Osteop.
144 Cloudesly Road
Islington
London N10EA, United Kingdom
Tel: +44 (0) 20 78 33 34 54
Fax: +44 (0) 20 78 33 34 54

Seminars and training courses in German and English

Reflex zone massage and therapy including crystal wands:

Ewald Kliegel
Rotenbergstrasse 154
D-70190 Stuttgart
Gemany
Tel: +49 (0)172 - 712 48 89
www.reflex-international.eu
info@reflex-international.eu

Lectures, seminars and advanced training in German and English for reflex zone therapy (therapeutic professions), professional reflex massage (for wellness professions and interested laypersons) and experiences with organ therapy – healing body and soul (for auto-experience). For up-to-date programmes of seminars and lecture information, see www.reflex-international.eu

Edition Cairn Elen

"After Elen had accomplished her wandering through the world, she placed a Cairn at the end of the Sarn Elen. Her path then led her back to the land between evening and morning. From this Cairn originated all stones that direct the way at crossroads up until today."*

(From a Celtic myth)

'Cairn Elen'** is the term used in Gaelic-speaking areas to refer to the ancient slab stones on track ways. They mark the spiritual paths, both the paths of the earth and that of knowledge.

These paths are increasingly falling into oblivion. Just as the old paths of the earth disappear under the modern asphalt streets, so also does certain ancient wisdom disappear under the data flood of modern information. For this reason, the desire and aim of the Edition Cairn Elen is to preserve ancient wisdom and link it with modern knowledge – for a flourishing future!

The Edition Cairn Elen in Neue Erde Verlag is published by Michael Gienger. The objective of the Edition is to present knowledge from research and tradition that has remained unpublished up until now. Areas of focus are nature, naturopathy and health, as well as consciousness and spiritual freedom.

Apart from current specialised literature, stories, fairytales, novels, lyric and artistic publications will also be published within the scope of Edition Cairn Elen. The knowledge thus transmitted reaches out not only to the intellect but also to the heart.

Contact
Edition Cairn Elen, Michael Gienger, Stäudach 58/1, D-72074 Tübingen
Tel: +49 (0)7071 - 364 719, Fax: +49 (0)7071 - 388 68,
eMail: buecher@michael-gienger.de, Website: www.michael-gienger.de

---

[1] Celtic 'cairn' [pronounced: carn] = 'Stone' (usually placed as an intentional shaped heap of stones), 'sarn' = 'Path', 'Elen, Helen' = 'Goddess of the Roads'

** Cairn Elen: in ancient and contemporary British culture, cairns are generally thought to be intentionally heaped piles of stones, rather than an individual stone such as a boulder or standing stone.

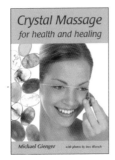

Michael Gienger
Crystal Massage for Health and Healing
112 Pages, full colour throughout, ISBN 978-1-84409-077-8

This book introduces a spectrum of massage possibilities using healing crystals. The techniques have been developed and refined by experts, and this wisdom is conveyed in simple and direct language, enhanced by photos. Any interested amateur will be amazed at the wealth of new therapeutic possibilities that open up when employing the healing power of crystals.

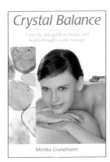

Monika Grundmann
Crystal Balance
A step-by-step guide to beauty and health through crystal massage
Paperback, full colour throughout, 112 pages,
ISBN 978-1-84409-132-4

Our physical wellbeing reflects every aspect of our lives and inner selves. As a result, massage is able to influence us on every level – mind, body and spirit.
    The Crystal Balance method aims to help our bodies relax and recover, encouraging our soul and spirit to 'bethemselves'. When we are truly 'ourselves', we are beautiful. It is as simple as that.

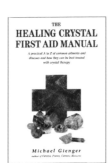

Michael Gienger
The Healing Crystal First Aid Manual
A practical A to Z of common ailments and illnesses and
how they can be best treated with crystal therapy
288 pages, with 16 colour plates, ISBN 978-1-84409-084-6

This is an easy-to-use A-Z guide for treating many common ailments and illnesses with the help of crystal therapy. It includes a comprehensive colour appendix with photographs and short descriptions of each gemstone recommended.

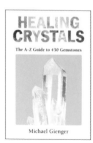

Michael Gienger
Healing Crystals
The A - Z Guide to 430 Gemstones
Paperback, 96 pages, ISBN 978-1-84409-067-9

All the important information about 430 healing gemstones in a neat pocket-book! Michael Gienger, known for his popular introductory work 'Crystal Power, Crystal Healing', here presents a comprehensive directory of all the gemstones currently in use. In a clear, concise and precise style, with pictures accompanying the text, the author describes the characteristics and healing functions of each crystal.

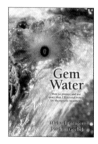

Michael Gienger, Joachim Goebel
Gem Water
How to prepare and use more than 130 crystal waters
for therapeutic treatments
Paperback, 96 pages, ISBN 978-1-84409-131-7

Adding crystals to water is both visually appealing and healthy. It is a known fact that water carries mineral information and Gem Water provides effective remedies, acting quickly on a physical level. It is similar and complementary to wearing crystals, but the effects are not necessarily the same.

Gem Water needs to be prepared and applied with care; this book explains everything you need to know to get started!

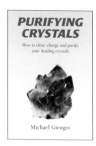

Michael Gienger
Purifying Crystals
How to clear, charge and purify your healing crystals
Paperback, full colour throughout, 64 pages, ISBN: 978-1-84409-147-8

Correct cleansing of crystals is an essential prerequisite for working with them successfully. But how can this be done effectively? There appear to be many different opinions on the subject. This useful little guidebook provides information about the known and less known methods for cleansing crystals, clearly illustrating which method is best for which aim, whether it be discharging, charging, cleansing on the outer level, cleansing on the energetic level, or elimination of attached information. Also included are step-by-step instructions for performing a crystal cleansing ceremony, and information about how to clear, cleanse and protect rooms with the help of crystals.

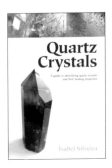

Isabel Silveira
Quartz Crystals
A guide to identifying quartz crystals and their healing properties
Paperback, full colour throughout, 80 pages,
ISBN 978-1-84409-148-5

This visually impressive book brings the reader up close to the beauty and diversity of the quartz crystal family. Its unique and concise presentation allows the reader to quickly and easily identify an array of quartz crystals and become familiar with their distinctive features and energetic properties.

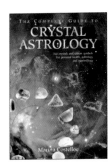

Marina Costelloe
The Complete Guide to Crystal Astrology
360 crystals and sabian symbols for personal health,
astrology and numerology
Paperback, 224 pages, full colour, with 360 pictures,
ISBN: 978-1-84409-103-4

Using this guide the reader will discover which of the 360 crystal elements is associated with the position of the sun at the time of their birth; learn about the relationship between birth charts, crystals, and planets; and find out how personal crystal elements are connected to numerology. The books also explores Marc Edmund Jones key words, Sabian symbols, and Jane Ridder-Patrick healing body points, ultimately teaching the readers how to reach a higher life potential.

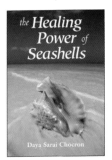

Daya Sarai Chocron
The Healing Power of Seashells
Paperback, 96 pages, ISBN: 978-1-84409-068-6

A quick guide to Seashells and their healing powers for everyone. This ancient Hawaiian wisdom is simple to understand and easy to put into practice. Included for your easy reference are photographs of Seashells and relevant descriptions to help you identify them. Most of the Seashells featured can befound on shores all over the world, and many are available for sale. This colourful book will immediately transport you to the beach!

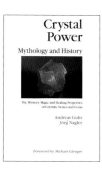

Andreas Guhr, Jörg Nagler
Crystal Power, Mythology and History
160pages, full colour throughout, ISBN: 978-1-84409-085-3

This book reveals the long- standing significance, high regard and use in therapy and healing of stones, crystals and gems – from the earliest civilizations such as Mesopotamia and Ancient Egypt, throughthe classical world of Greece and Rome and into medieval European cultures. In addition, there is acomprehensive Appendix, in which minerals and crystals are listed with their respective mineralogical,historical, astrological and healing properties.

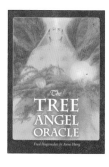

Fred Hageneder, Anne Heng
The Tree Angel Oracle
36 colour cards (95 x 133 mm) plus book, 112 pages,
ISBN: 978-1-84409-078-5

There are two types of angels: those with wings, and those with leaves. For thousands of years, those seeking advice or wanting to give thanks to Mother Nature have walked the ancient paths into the sacred grove. Because today sacred groves have become scarcer, and venerable old trees in tranquil spots are hard to find when we need them, Earthdancer is pleased to present this tree oracle to bring the tree angels closer to us all once more.

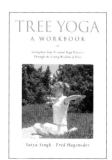

Satya Singh and Fred Hageneder
Tree Yoga: a Workbook
Strengthen Your Personal Yoga Practice
Through the Living Wisdom of Trees
Paperback two colours, 224 pages,ISBN: 978-1-84409-119-5

Revealing the dynamic bond between man and tree, this inspired yoga handbook offers a detailed review of the ancient wisdom of Kundalini Yoga and unveils the inner power of trees, as well as their unique characteristics and energies. Yoga exercises based on this wisdom are provided, each of which operates by fostering a connection with the inner essence of a different tree, from birch and lime to elm and rowan. With full illustrations and step-by-step instructions.

Publisher's Note

The information in this volume has been compiled according to the best of our knowledge and belief, and the healing properties of the crystals have been tested many times over. However, bearing in mind that people react in different ways, neither the publisher nor the author can give guarantee for the effectiveness or safety of the use or application in individual cases. In cases of serious health problems, please consult your doctor or naturopath.

Crystal Wands
Ewald Kliegel

First Edition 2009

This English edition © 2009 Earthdancer GmbH

English translation © 2008 Astrid Mick

Editorial: Claudine Bloomfield

Originally published in German as
Massagen mit Edelsteingriffeln
World © Neue Erde GmbH, Saarbruecken, Germany
All rights reserved

Title page: photo Ines Blersch
Design: Dragon Design UK Ltd.
Typesetting and graphics: Dragon Design UK Ltd.
Typeset in Garamond Itc Light Condensed

Entire production: Midas Printing

Printed and bound in China

ISBN 978-1-84409-152-2

Published by Earthdancer GmbH, an imprint of:
Findhorn Press, 305a The Park, Findhorn,
Forres, IV36 3TE, Great Britain
www.earthdancer.co.uk
www.findhornpress.com

EARTHDANCER
A FINDHORN PRESS IMPRINT
For further information and book catalogue contact:
Findhorn Press, 305a The Park, Forres, IV36 3TE, Scotland.
Earthdancer Books is an imprint of Findhorn Press.
tel +44 (0)1309-690582, fax +44 (0)131 777 2711

info@findhornpress.com, www.earthdancer.co.uk, www.findhornpress.com

For more information on crystal healing visit www.crystalhealingbooks.com

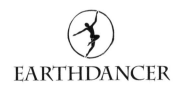

A FINDHORN PRESS IMPRINT